Shedding Light
on
Genetically Engineered Food

Shedding Light on Genetically Engineered Food

What You Don't Know About the Food You're Eating and What You Can Do to Protect Yourself

Beth H. Harrison, Ph.D.

iUniverse, Inc.
New York Lincoln Shanghai

Shedding Light on Genetically Engineered Food
What You Don't Know About the Food You're Eating and What You Can Do to Protect Yourself

iUniverse books may be ordered through booksellers or by contacting:

iUniverse
2021 Pine Lake Road, Suite 100
Lincoln, NE 68512
www.iuniverse.com
1-800-Authors (1-800-288-4677)

Because of the dynamic nature of the Internet, any Web addresses or links contained in this book may have changed since publication and may no longer be valid.

The views expressed in this work are solely those of the author and do not necessarily reflect the views of the publisher, and the publisher hereby disclaims any responsibility for them.

ISBN: 978-0-595-45180-7 (pbk)
ISBN: 978-0-595-69326-9 (cloth)
ISBN: 978-0-595-89488-8 (ebk)

Printed in the United States of America

This book is dedicated to my best friend and husband Jeff. Your incredible support and encouragement made this journey possible. Words cannot express my immense gratitude for all you do and who you are. My appreciation also goes to Sasha and Riley—your patience and understanding have been extraordinary. Thanks for the encouragement. I am so fortunate to have you all in my life.

My gratitude also goes to all of the people who are working to bring the topic of GE food to light, and to the individuals who assisted me during my research. Thank you so much, Jeffrey Smith, for taking time out of your busy schedule to communicate at length with me via email, which began in 2005. I also appreciate your granting me permission to reprint the 2006 *Scientists' Open Letter* and the excerpt from your latest book *Genetic Roulette*. To Dr. Arpad Pusztai, your work and dedication to real science is inspiring. Thank you for your encouragement and for your permission to reprint the 2006 *Scientists' Open Letter*. Dr. David Suzuki, I appreciate your permission to quote the insightful "Biotechnology: A Geneticist's Perspective." And thank you Dr. Mae-Wan Ho for allowing me to quote your material from the Institute of Science in Society Web site. Brian Tokar, director of the Biotechnology Project at Vermont's Institute for Social Ecology, and Richard Caplan, with U.S. Public Interest Research Group, thank you for your help when I began researching this material. My thanks also go to Joseph Mendelson, legal director for the Center for Food Safety, for your assistance regarding CFS's lawsuit against the FDA, and to United Nation's Environmental Program's legal officer Worku Damena Yifru for your correspondence regarding the Cartagena Protocol on Biosafety.

Contents

Introduction
Americans Kept in the Dark

Monsanto should not have to vouchsafe the safety of biotech food. Our interest is in selling as much of it as possible. Assuring its safety is the FDA's job.[1]
Philip Angell, while director of corporate communications at Monsanto, quoted in the New York Times, October 25, 1998

Ultimately, it is the food producer who is responsible for assuring safety.[2]
FDA Statement of Food Policy: Foods Derived from New Plant Varieties, May 29, 1992 Federal Register

Food today is big business—a business of money and politics. It has simply become a commodity to be patented, owned, and sold on the global market. No independent, peer-reviewed scientific proof exists of the safety of humans consuming genetically engineered (GE) food.

Because there is no labeling of GE food in America, you have been part of a large-scale genetic experiment *without your knowledge or consent.* While the U.S. government protects multinational biotechnology corporations' interests, who is watching out for you?

Some people might say, "Why should I care if I eat GE food? If it weren't safe, the Food and Drug Administration (FDA) and the U.S. Department of Agriculture (USDA) would not allow it in the food supply." However, after reading this book, you might rethink that assumption, and here are a few reasons why:

- no GE food has ever been safety-tested for human consumption;

- manufacturers can introduce a GE food without informing the government or consumers;

- largely due to biotech lobbying, GE food is not required to be labeled in the U.S. as they are in other countries, even though polls have overwhelmingly shown that the majority of American consumers want GE labeling;

- scientists have warned about potential health risks of consuming GE food, including cancers and other illnesses;

- children face the greatest risk from the potential dangers of GE food because their bodies develop at a fast pace and are more likely to be influenced and show the adverse effects from it; and

- insurance companies will not insure the biotechnology industry because it is too risky.

You might assume the U.S. government would do everything to ensure that GE food is safe for consumers and the environment. As one of the U.S. regulatory agencies, the FDA's mission is to protect public health. So where does the FDA stand on the safety of GE food? The agency asserted in the 1992 *Statement of Food Policy: Foods Derived from New Plant Varieties* that the food producer is responsible for safety: "FDA has not found it necessary to conduct comprehensive scientific reviews of foods derived from bioengineered plants … Ultimately, it is the food producer who is responsible for assuring safety."[3, 4]

According to biotech-giant Monsanto's former director of corporate communications, "Monsanto should not have to vouchsafe the safety of biotech food. Our interest is in selling as much of it as possible. Assuring its safety is the FDA's job."[5]

So, if neither the U.S. government nor the U.S. food producers are responsible for the safety of GE food, *who is?*

The biotech industry often claims that the safety of GE products has been certified through a rigorous approval process carried out by the FDA. In reality, GE crops are only subject to *voluntary* consultations with companies that choose to consult with the agency about their products. Because the consultations are voluntary, the FDA does not require specific safety studies or test methods to be conducted. The agency accepts summaries of whatever testing the company has chosen to do; however, summaries are not required, either.

Few valid safety animal studies have been conducted on GE food, and no adequate tests have been performed on biochemistry, immunology, tissue pathology, gut function, liver function, and kidney function. Animal-feeding studies have also been too short to test for many illnesses and effects in the next generation.[6] Scientific studies have revealed that some animals fed GE food developed potentially pre-cancerous cell growth; smaller brains, livers, and testicles; damaged immune systems; partial atrophy of the liver; lesions in the livers, stomachs, and kidneys; inflammation of the kidneys; and problems with their blood cells. These concerns have not been followed-up on or accounted for.[7] It is naïve to expect companies that stand to gain financially to offer information voluntarily when it could jeopardize lucrative products.

As far as U.S. regulatory agencies are concerned, if a biotech company says its products are safe, that is enough for approval.

Dr. Ignacio Chapela, assistant professor of microbial ecology, Department of Environmental Science, Policy, and Management at the University of California at Berkeley, pointed out, "We have started seeing pieces of DNA interacting with each other in ways that are entirely unpredictable. I think this is probably the largest biological experiment humanity has ever entered into."[8]

So why has the majority of the American public never heard about GE food and the potential health risks?

The FDA's decision not to require labeling has played an important role in keeping most Americans in the dark regarding the GE food they are eating. At the same time, people in the rest of the world seem to be more informed, and their governments have taken action to ban or label it. As of 2005, more than forty countries, including the European Union (EU), Russia, the Czech Republic, Japan, South Korea, Taiwan, Australia, New Zealand and Ecuador, have laws requiring the labeling of GE food.[9] Such labeling is going on worldwide, giving citizens in those countries information about GE food and the freedom to choose *not* to eat it.

Since 1994, GE food has been force-fed to millions of American infants, children, and adults every day. Because the United States and Canada are the only industrialized countries in the world without a GE labeling law, most citizens do not even know they have been consuming GE food. According to the Pew Initiative on Food and Biotechnology poll released in December 2006, 60% of Americans believed they had never eaten GE food and 14% said they did not know if they had ever consumed it.[10]

In reality, GE food is sold daily in the United States without identifying labels. These include soy, cotton, corn, canola oil, dairy products, summer squash, potatoes, tomatoes, radicchio, and papayas, as well as other fruits and vegetables. This altered food is also used in up to 75% of processed food products, such as frozen and microwave foods, sodas, fast foods, baking mixes and baked goods, breakfast cereals, snack foods, sauces, margarine, salad dressings, and even baby food and infant formula.

It has to make you wonder. If the majority of processed food in America is genetically altered, yet consumers do not benefit from eating it, why are they eating it?

According to the Biotechnology Industry Organization's (BIO) Web site (the industry's largest trade organization), the biotech industry is a multi-billion dollar industry whose goal is simply "to build revenue and a profit-generating business." The first decade of planting the billionth acre of GE crops occurred in 2005 with a global market worth about $6.15 billion in 2006. While there has been growth around the world, the global agricultural biotechnology market remains dominated by Missouri-based Monsanto.[11]

It is no coincidence that the largest biotechnology companies are the world's largest herbicide and pesticide companies. While some GE crops have been created to produce pesticides in each one of their cells, the majority of GE crops were created to tolerate large doses of a particular company's weed killers or pesticides. These so-called "life science" companies alter and patent their seeds, requiring farmers to repurchase them yearly, and ensure that crops cannot be grown without their patented chemicals.

Government support for biotech crops seems to stem from two important facts: they are U.S.-developed, and biotech companies have made significant financial contributions to politicians and political parties. For instance, Monsanto paid more than $22.5 million in lobbying money from 1999 to 2004.[12]

With billions of dollars at stake, the U.S. government and the biotechnology industry have kept the American public uninformed about GE food and its risks. Food labeling is essential for a consumer's right to know. The FDA currently labels irradiated food, organic produce, processed food methods such as "grown without pesticides or preservatives," and allows kosher symbols on certain foods. These labels provide consumers with information, yet biotech proponents contend that labeling GE food would "confuse" people, even though polls have overwhelmingly concluded that the majority of the population wants GE labeling.

The article *Why Biotech Labeling Can Confuse Consumers*, written by the Council for Biotechnology Information (CBI), states that because the FDA considers biotech food "substantially equivalent" to conventional food, labeling biotech food "could sow confusion among consumers." However, CBI's real concern was revealed when the article declared, "Ninety-two percent of food industry leaders, for example, believe that mandatory biotech food labeling ... will instead be perceived as a 'warning' by at least some consumers."[13] CBI is an industry organization dedicated to promoting biotechnology in agriculture.

How have the biotech industry and the U.S. government tried to sell the public on the necessity of genetically altered food?

The biotech industry and the U.S. government have methodically promised a variety of benefits: more nutrition, better flavor, higher crop yields, fewer pesticides, longer shelf life, and more. Actually, GE crops have failed to deliver benefits, while consumers continue to assume all of the health risks.

Proponents have even claimed GE food is necessary to increase food production to "feed the world." But claiming that GE crops are necessary to feed the world is only plausible if it is mistakenly assumed that people go hungry because there is a shortage of food. On the contrary, food overproduction is a problem today, yet people in third-world countries are so poor that they cannot afford to buy what is already grown.

The future of the world's food supply should be based upon sound science, not on propaganda of corporations with high-priced public relations and marketing budgets. History has shown that many of the same biotechnology companies that tell the public to trust them with the world's food supply *have repeatedly done business at the expense of public health.*

The empty promises made by the U.S. government and the biotechnology industry cannot obscure the fact that there has never been evidence of the safety of consuming GE food. Americans are risking their health for the corporate bottom line. Until they have been independently tested and found safe, any foods that contain GE ingredients should be clearly labeled. Citizens in other countries have a choice *not* to eat GE food thanks to labeling. Why should Americans be denied the freedom to make an equally informed choice?

Chapter 1
The Biotech Façade

These companies are going into the seed banks to find seeds that have not been patented and patent them. Then they can take their patented seeds and replace existing ones and own the marketplace.[1]
Andrew Kimbrell, executive director for Center for Food Safety, quoted in Deborah Garcia's The Future of Food documentary

Those of us in the industry can take comfort ... after all, we're the technical experts. We know we're right. The "anti's" obviously don't understand the science and are just as obviously pushing a hidden agenda, probably to destroy capitalism.[2]
Robert B. Shapiro, Monsanto's former CEO, quoted in John Robbins' The Food Revolution

When GE food was introduced in America more than a decade ago, it was promoted as a solution to the world's food problems; however, those benefits have never been realized. In fact, scientific studies have shown that GE food poses serious risks to humans, animals, and wildlife. Human health effects of consuming GE food can include toxic and allergic reactions, antibiotic resistance, immune suppression, and cancers. As for the environment, in some cases, massive chemicals have been needed because GE crops are developing resistance to some companies' herbicides. Just as concerning is the irreversible contamination of non-GE life forms with GE material.[3]

PRECARIOUS BREEDING

Deoxyribonucleic acid (DNA) is the blueprint for organisms that controls biochemical processes such as life, growth, and physical characteristics. The segments of DNA associated with specific functions of an organism are called genes. Combining genes from different species is known as recombinant DNA technology, and the resulting organism is said to be "genetically modified" (GM), "genetically engineered" (GE), or "transgenic." Genetically modified organisms (GMOs) are the actual organisms created through genetic engineering and are terms commonly used on labels such as "non-GMO" or "GMO-free." Biotechnology, the interaction of biology with technology, is the manipulation of organisms on a molecular level to knowingly create, develop, and market a variety of products.

To date, only about 3-5% of DNA function is understood, while the other 95-97% has been referred to as "junk DNA," or molecular garbage, by some molecular biologists because they have been unable to determine its function.[4] Most DNA knowledge is about structural genes responsible for body structures, which are the simplest parts of the system, but the genetic code of regulator genes is hardly known. Without understanding 95-97% of DNA function, no one can rationally claim to foresee and control the effects of genetically engineered food.

The commercialization of GE organisms is a relatively new national industry. Crossing the species barrier to create new life forms is something that has never occurred in nature and is not an extension of conventional breeding. For example, scientists have created potatoes with bacteria genes, "super pigs and sheep" that have been crossed with human growth genes, fish with cow growth genes, tomatoes with flounder genes, rice with human hormone genes, and thousands of other new, unnatural creations.

The biotech industry claims that genetic engineering is precise and safe, but when genetic material is inserted into a new host, uncertainty always exists. Living organisms are not machines with interchangeable parts. Individual genes do not have a one-to-one correspondence with certain desired characteristics or traits. Gene "splicing" is imprecise and unpredictable.[5] Scientist Dr. David Suzuki, world-renowned geneticist, academic, and author of more than thirty books, wrote in *Biotechnology: A Geneticist's Perspective*, "Reductionism is a scientific method that focuses on parts to understand the whole of a mechanistic universe; however, regarding genetics, physicists learned early in the last century that parts interact synergistically so that new properties emerge from their combination that could not be anticipated from their individual properties."[6]

Likewise, Richard Strohman, eminent scientist and former chair of the Department of Molecular and Cell Biology at Berkeley, stated the problem with GE food this way: "Genes exist in networks—interactive networks which have a logic of their own … And the fact that the industry folks don't deal with these networks is what makes their science incomplete and dangerous … Biotechnologists assume all pieces of DNA can be removed and inserted as if they are equivalent, but genes don't exist independently; they exist within complex, synergistic sets of networks."[7]

Two common methods of gene insertion are used to create GE seeds, and both result in mutations. The first method uses *Agrobacterium* bacteria (a genus of bacteria that causes tumors in plants), which contain pieces of DNA called plasmids. One section of this plasmid creates tumors, and genetic engineers replace the tumor-creating section of the plasmid with one or more genes. They then use the altered *Agrobacterium* to infect a plant's DNA with those foreign genes.[8]

Another method of gene insertion is to shoot DNA through the cell walls of a target organism. A gene gun penetrates the cell walls with bacteria and viruses to invade the host. However, where the trait will land in the target organism is unknown. Therefore, when the gene gun is fired, scientists have little idea where the desired traits will crash through the cell walls and can end up creating imbalances, such as erratic expression, turning on or off genes, and other potential problems.

Director of the Institute for Responsible Technology and author of the internationally best-selling book on GE food *Seeds of Deception,* Jeffrey M. Smith pointed out a misconception regarding GE food in his recent book *Genetic Roulette: The Documented Health Risks of Genetically Engineered Foods:*

> The prevailing worldview behind the development of GM foods was that genes were like Lego blocks—independent pieces that snap into place. This is false. The process of creating a GM crop can produce massive changes in the natural functioning of the plant's DNA. Native genes can be mutated, deleted, or permanently turned off or on, and hundreds may change their levels of expression. The inserted gene can become truncated, fragmented, mixed with other genes, inverted or multiplied, and the GM protein it produces may have unintended characteristics with harmful side effects.
>
> To make this clear, we'll use the popular analogy comparing DNA to a book. The four bases that make up the genetic sequence are the letters in the book; the genes are special pages that describe characters called proteins.
>
> The common way people explain and promote genetic engineering is to say, "It is just like taking a page out of one book and putting it into another."
>
> In reality, a book would look quite different after it had undergone genetic engineering. The inserted page (gene) may turn out to be multiple identical pages, partial pages, or small bits of text. Sections of the insert are misspelled, deleted, inverted, or scrambled. Next to the inserts, the story is often indecipherable, with random letters, new text, and pages missing.
>
> The rest of the book has also changed. There are now typos throughout, sometimes hundreds or thousands of them. Letters are switched, words are scrambled, and sentences are deleted, repeated, or reversed.
>
> Passages from one part of the book, even whole chapters (chromosomes), may be relocated or repeated elsewhere, and bits of text from entirely different books can show up from time-to-time. Many of the characters in the story (proteins) now act differently. Some minor roles have become prominent, leads have been demoted, and some may have switched roles from hero to villain or vice versa.

And, if you get bored with this story, take the original book, insert another page—even the same one—and the changes will be completely different. Or stick with the original book, and over time, it might actually rearrange the inserted page.[9]

Nature is unpredictable. Perceptions about what genes are, how they work, and what scientists know about genes is constantly changing. And given the fact that 95-97% of DNA function is hardly known, how can the biotechnology industry and the U.S. government claim with certainty that genetically engineering the world's food supply is understood, predictable, and safe for human consumption?

Molecular biologist and professor in the Division of Natural Sciences at the State University of New York at Purchase, Dr. Leibe Cavalieri said it is "simplistic, if not downright simple-minded, to claim that genetic engineering is substantially the same as traditional breeding, and doing so borders on sham."[10] Dr. Cavalieri has written extensively on biotechnology issues.

PATENTING AND OWNING LIFE

Humanity's "commons" are what we all need to live: water, air, land, the forests and the oceans, our genes, our food sources, wildlife, and ecosystems. The commons are what we hold in trust for future generations, yet none of us owns them. Seeds have always been an important part of the commons, but biotech corporations create their own patented GE seeds to be bought and sold on the global market.

There have always been laws against patenting life. But in 1971, a General Electric Company microbiologist challenged those laws and applied to the U.S. Patent and Trademark Office (PTO) to patent a transgenic microorganism that would consume oil spills in the ocean. The PTO rejected the patent request, saying that living things are not patentable under U.S. patent law. However, that PTO decision was taken to the Court of Customs and Patent Appeals, where General Electric won by a three-to-two decision. The majority of the court agreed that "the fact that microorganisms ... are alive is without legal significance."[11]

The PTO then appealed that decision and took the case to the U.S. Supreme Court. In 1980, the Supreme Court justices ruled in favor of General Electric's microbiologist, granting a patent on the first GE life form. Justice William Brennan said it "is the role of Congress, not this court, to broaden or narrow the reach of patent laws."[12] Seven years later in 1987, the PTO reversed its earlier position against patents on life and issued a ruling that all GE living organisms, including animals, are potentially patentable.[13] Private companies were then assured that they could invest in GE research without worrying about their "inventions" being copied without financial compensation.

Author and president of the Foundation on Economic Trends, Jeremy Rifkin said in his book *The Biotech Century: Harnessing the Gene and Remaking the World* that it was that very decision that laid the legal groundwork for the privatization of the genetic commons. He also pointed out that it was "soon thereafter that chemical, pharmaceutical, and biotech companies sped up their research and development work, knowing that patent protection meant the opportunity to own the genetic commons for commercial gain in the years ahead."[14]

WHO IS MESSING WITH YOUR FOOD?

Multinational chemical companies, some of the worst polluters of the twentieth century, have attempted to remake themselves into "life sciences" companies by modifying seeds for food crops. They alter seeds to be resistant to some of their most profitable chemical products, patent the seeds, and then force-feed GE foods derived from the altered seeds to an unsuspecting public. All along, they have been claiming their new GE foods are safe, just as they have done in the past with their dangerous chemicals.[15] On the surface, this may appear not to be a cause for concern, except for the fact that GE foods have never been proven safe for human consumption.

It has always been an individual's choice to avoid these multinational companies' chemicals for gardening or yard work, but everyone has to eat. Without labeling, however, consumers have no choice but to eat these experimental products.

"By the 1990s, corporations began patenting not only GMO seeds but also seeds that hadn't been genetically engineered. The only requirement was that they hadn't been patented before," said Andrew Kimbrell, public-interest attorney, activist, author, and executive director of the Center for Food Safety. "These companies are going into the seed banks to find seeds that have not been patented and patent them. Then they can take their patented seeds and replace existing ones and own the marketplace."[16]

Just four companies—Monsanto, Syngenta, Bayer, and DuPont—control the majority of the world's GE crops. The following are just some examples of how these companies *have hugely profited at the expense of public health.* And for more than a decade, they have been reprogramming the DNA of much of the world's food supply without public debate.

Monsanto

Monsanto is currently the world's top producer of GE seeds; the overwhelming majority of all GE crops grown worldwide come from Monsanto technology.[17] With a history of unleashing products that have proven to be devastating to people and the environment, Monsanto, founded as a chemical company in 1901, says its GE food is safe for human consumption.

Agent Orange

Monsanto's herbicide 2,4,5-T contained a highly toxic chemical byproduct, the potent dioxin TCDD. This herbicide was one of two chemicals used in Agent Orange, a defoliant used by the U.S. military in the Vietnam War. Monsanto was not the only company that produced Agent Orange, but its products contained the highest levels of dioxin. The negative health effects of exposure to Agent Orange have been documented over the past thirty-plus years, and it is considered one of the most toxic chemicals on the planet, causing everything from severe birth defects, cancers, and neurological disorders, to death.[18]

However, Monsanto continues to deny that the banned chemical is toxic and refuses any responsibility in compensating American Vietnam War veterans and civilians who have been harmed by exposure to Agent Orange.

Dioxin Cover-Up

In the 1980s, a $16-million-damage award against Monsanto revealed that many of Monsanto's products, from household herbicides to the Santophen germicide once used in Lysol brand disinfectant, were knowingly contaminated with dioxin. A review by Dr. Cate Jenkins of the Environmental Protection Agency's (EPA) Regulatory Development Branch documented a systematic record of fraudulent science, where Monsanto knowingly submitted false information to the EPA.

In her November 1990 report, *Criminal Investigation of Monsanto Corporation—Cover-up of Dioxin Contamination in Products, Falsification of Dioxin Health Studies*, Jenkins cited internal Monsanto documents that revealed the company doctored samples of herbicides that were submitted, hid evidence regarding the contamination of Lysol, and excluded several hundred of its sickest former employees from its comparative health studies.[19]

Roundup

Roundup brand of seeds are engineered to tolerate high doses of Monsanto's best-selling product, the toxic weed killer Roundup (glyphosate). The U.S. Fish and Wildlife Service has identified that it endangers seventy-four plant species, kills fish, impedes the growth of earthworms and increases their mortality, is toxic to soil microbes, and is the third most commonly reported cause of all forms of pesticide-related illness in California.[20]

A study by eminent Swedish oncologists Dr. Lennart Hardell and Dr. Mikael Eriksson revealed links between glyphosate and non-Hodgkin's lymphoma, a form of cancer. The American Academy of Family Physicians' epidemiological research has also linked exposure to the herbicide with increased risk of non-Hodgkin's lymphoma.[21] The June 2005 scientific journal *Environmental Health Perspectives* reported that glyphosate damages human placental cells at exposure levels ten times less than what Monsanto claims is safe,[22] while a study in the August 2005 journal *Ecological Applications* found that even when applied at concentrations that are one-third of the maximum concentrations typically found in waterways, Roundup still killed up to 71% of tadpoles in the study.[23]

Despite these studies, Monsanto advertises Roundup, sprayed heavily on GE crops around the world, as one of the safest pesticides on the market.

Posilac

Also known as recombinant bovine growth hormone (rBGH) or recombinant bovine somatotropin (rBST), this synthetic GE hormone is injected into a cow's pituitary gland every two weeks, resulting in an increased milk output by up to 20%.[24]

Posilac-injected cows produce milk with high levels of insulin-like growth factor-1 (IGF-1), a cancer-promoter in humans. Since 1994, every industrialized country in the world—except the United States—has banned rBGH milk. The Codex Alimentarius Commission, an international food standards body, which is a joint venture of the Food and Agriculture Organization of the United Nations and the World Health Organization, refuses to certify that rBGH is safe; even the World Trade Organization has refused to endorse Monsanto's claim that rBGH is safe for use in the dairy supply.[25]

Ironically, because there is already an overproduction of milk in the United States, taxpayers pay more than $300 million each year[26] just to buy the surplus milk to subsidize the industry and dairy prices.

Terminator Technology

For centuries, farmers have saved seeds from each crop to be able to plant them for their crop the following year. But Monsanto, one of the companies claiming GE crops are to help feed the world, developed a "technology protection system" that renders seeds sterile after one planting. This technology obligates farmers to return to Monsanto every year to buy new seeds.

Commonly known as "terminator technology," it was developed by the USDA and Delta & Pine Land Company (now owned by Monsanto) with taxpayer funding.

Polychlorinated Biphenyls (PCBs)

Monsanto has produced or granted production licenses for most of the world's PCBs. Used for various industrial purposes, PCBs are toxic environmental pollutants that accumulate in animal and human tissues.

In 2002, Monsanto was found guilty of releasing tons of PCBs into the city of Anniston, Alabama, and covering it up for years. Anniston residents did not learn about the pollution until 1996, even though Monsanto's internal company documents from the 1960s stated, "CONFIDENTIAL: Read and Destroy." Apparently, Monsanto knew about the dangers of PCBs but wanted to protect its PCB monopoly, regardless of health or environmental risks.[27]

For example, in 1966, Monsanto managers discovered that "fish placed in a local creek turned belly-up within ten seconds, spurting blood and shedding skin as if dunked into boiling acid." In 1969, they found a fish in another creek with 7,500 times the legal PCB level, but never told anyone and concluded that, "there is little object in going to expensive extremes in limiting discharges. We can't afford to lose one dollar of business." [28] A committee that Monsanto formed to address controversies about PCBs had two objectives: *to permit continued sales and profits and to protect the image of the corporation.*

Monsanto stopped making PCBs in Anniston in 1971, and in 1976, PCBs were banned as a cancer-causing carcinogen with enactment of the Toxic Substances Control Act. Even so, documents show that for more than two decades after ending production, Monsanto withheld disturbing information about the contamination in Anniston.

Finally, in February 2002, Monsanto was charged with "negligence, wantonness, suppression of truth, nuisance, trespass, and outrage." Under Alabama law, the charge of outrage requires conduct "… so outrageous in character and extreme in degree as to go beyond all possible bounds of decency so as to be regarded as atrocious and intolerable in civilized society."[29] Monsanto lost a series of court decisions, resulting in $700 million in damages that were awarded to thousands of residents of Anniston.

Bribery

In January 2005, the U.S. Securities and Exchange Commission charged Monsanto with violating the Foreign Corrupt Practices Act. To test GE crops illegally in Indonesia, Monsanto bribed more than 140 Indonesian government officials and their families with an amount totaling more than $700,000 between 1997 and 2002. Monsanto agreed to pay a $1 million penalty to defer prosecution charges by the U.S. Department of Justice.[30]

While these historical perspectives provide examples of Monsanto's corporate activities, its shift in focus toward the public food supply raises serious concerns.

Consolidating the Food Chain

Monsanto has been advancing the use of genetic engineering in agriculture by taking control of many of the largest, most established seed companies in the United States. The company once gained its wealth almost exclusively through agricultural chemicals, but for more than a decade they spent approximately $10 billion buying seed producers and companies in other sectors of the agricultural business. In 2005, they bought Seminis, the biggest producer of vegetable seeds in the world.[31]

"What you are seeing is not just a consolidation of seed companies; it's really a consolidation of the entire food chain," commented Robert Fraley, co-president of Monsanto's agricultural sector in 1996.[32]

Monsanto vs U.S. Farmers

In January 2005, the Center for Food Safety (CFS) released a report about Monsanto's abuse of the U.S. patent law to control crop seeds. Farmers whose non-GE crops are contaminated due to blow-over by GE crops can be sued for patent infringement and technology fees, forcing farmers into bankruptcy. As Andrew Kimbrell put it, "These lawsuits are nothing less than corporate extortion of American farmers. Monsanto is polluting American farms with its genetically engineered crops, not properly informing farmers about these altered seeds, and then profiting from its own irresponsibility and negligence by suing innocent farmers ..."[33]

According to a CFS report, in 2004, Monsanto filed ninety lawsuits against American farmers in twenty-five states, which involved 147 farmers and thirty-nine small businesses or farm companies. Monsanto has an annual budget of $10 million and a staff of seventy-five devoted solely to investigating and prosecuting farmers. "Monsanto would like nothing more than to be the sole source for staple crop seeds in this country and around the world," said Joseph Mendelson, CFS legal director. "And it will aggressively overturn centuries-old farming practices and drive its own clients out of business through lawsuits to achieve this goal."[34]

Monsanto's New Invention: The Pig

Monsanto is trying to patent pig-breeding techniques and claim the animals born as a result belong to them. Consumer activists warn that if Monsanto is permitted pig-related patents, its control over agriculture could be unprecedented. "We're afraid that Monsanto and other big companies are getting control of the world's genetic resources," said Christoph Then, a patent expert with Greenpeace in Germany.[35] There have been hundreds of animal patents granted in the past, but the majority of them are GE animals used for laboratory research, not the average farm animal.

Syngenta

This company was formed by a merger of the crop biotech units of the Swiss company Novartis, which resulted from the merger of chemical and pharmaceutical giants Ciba-Geigy and Sandoz, and AstraZeneca (Astra was a Swedish pharmaceutical company, and Zeneca was formerly the pharmaceutical and agrochemical unit of Britain's Imperial Chemical Industries). Syngenta is the world's number-one pesticide maker and number-one biotech patent holder. It owns Advanta, one of the world's largest seed producers, as well as other major seed firms.[36]

Golden Rice

Syngenta created Golden Rice, a GE strain of rice that was touted as producing high levels of beta-carotene to overcome vitamin-A deficiency, especially helping third-world countries. Announced in January 2000, when much of the world was first rejecting GE foods, Golden Rice promised to save millions of people from blindness and disease.

Syngenta claimed it had no economic interest in the project, yet in 2004, the company filed patents for Golden Rice in more than one hundred countries, including India, China, Indonesia, the Philippines, and several African countries. The patent applications reveal that the company's humanitarianism was really about commercial interests, since there is no reason to file a patent except to make money from it.

Golden Rice, however, would not save the world from malnutrition. It produced so little beta-carotene that a woman would need to eat nearly twenty pounds of cooked Golden Rice every day, and a child would need twelve pounds in order to get sufficient vitamin A. According to Dr. Vandana Shiva, a New Delhi-based physicist, environmental activist, and author of more than three hundred papers in leading scientific and technical journals, "Golden Rice is about public relations for an industry facing problems; it's a hoax and not truly about feeding starving people."[37]

Adrian Dubock, head of biotechnology ventures and licensing at Syngenta in Europe, commented, "Biotechnology industry representatives ... held Golden Rice up as a model for the way genetically modified crops could help feed the world. It was a badly needed positive message for an industry under fire ... Amid the controversy about genetically engineered food, Golden Rice was a brilliant flash—something slick U.S. marketing firms could sell to a skeptical public in television and print ads."[38]

Terminator Technology

In 2001, Syngenta announced that it applied to test their "terminator technology" in an open field trial in England. "Terminator technology" created sterile seeds, and in this case, would render seeds sterile unless Syngenta's own chemical was applied. A letter from its research and development director in February 1999 stated, "We are not developing any system that would stop farmers growing second-generation seed, nor do we have any intention of doing so." However, the application to test the technology showed that Syngenta is working on a plant that will not survive to a second generation or even grow successfully during a first generation without the company's chemicals applied to it.[39]

Bt Corn Contamination

Reuters reported in March 2005 that Syngenta said it mistakenly sold to farmers an experimental Bt "pesticidal" corn seed, which was approved for animal feed only. Hundreds of tons of the unapproved corn were planted in open fields in the United States from 2001 to 2004 before Syngenta acknowledged the mistake; however, no recalls for the corn were planned because a Syngenta representative claimed the corn posed no health or environmental risks.

"It shows that regulators and the industry can't be trusted to keep genetically engineered organisms from contaminating the food supply," said Greg Jaffe, biotech director for the nonprofit Center for Science in the Public Interest in Washington, D.C.[40]

As a result, in 2005, the EU voted to ban all imports of corn feed from the United States unless the shipments are accompanied with an analytical report from an accredited lab that guarantees the contents do not include any of that type of GE corn. Germany's Consumer Protection Minister Renate Kuenast said that Europe had no choice but to ban GE corn from the United States because American farmers had no system in place for labeling GE seeds and tracing them back to their producers. "The ban is the only possible way of dealing with such an unbelievable sloppiness! In the U.S., unlike Europe, GE food isn't labeled, and it can't be traced back to the producer ... There is a lack of transparency."[41]

Syngenta agreed to pay a $375,000 fine, but the EU corn ban costs Americans up to $450 million a year in lost revenues from export shipments.

Mega Patents

In an August 2005 press release from Swissaid, a non-governmental organization, Tina Goethe said Syngenta took a step closer to controlling the food supply by filing fifteen patent applications on several thousands of gene sequences from rice and other important crop plants. "With these patents, Syngenta is claiming the work of breeders and farmers from the past centuries as the company's own invention. The attempt to monopolize thousands of gene sequences from the most important crop plants in one rush is nothing less than a theft of common goods."[42]

By claiming the genetic information of rice, the company's goal is to own all similar gene sequences in any other useful plants, enabling Syngenta and other companies to determine prices and access to all kinds of seeds. According to Francois Meienberg from Berne Declaration in Switzerland, "These patents must never be granted. If the company follows its claims, they should expect public protests and legal actions against it. Politicians should initiate a legal framework to stop companies such as Syngenta, Monsanto, DuPont, and Bayer to gain control on genetic resources."[43]

Bayer CropScience

Bayer CropScience, a unit of the German company Bayer AG, became a leading GE crop producer with its purchase of Aventis in 2001. Aventis brought to Bayer the formerly independent Belgian biotech company Plant Genetic Systems, India's ProAgro, and Nunhems (Sunseeds in North America), which is the world's fourth-largest vegetable-seed producer. With the Aventis buyout, Bayer became the world's number-two pesticide maker, after Syngenta.[44]

Star Link and Liberty Link

Star Link corn, a GE corn created to act like a pesticide, was approved for use as animal feed, but not for human consumption. In 2000, consumers reported severe allergic reactions to some corn products, and subsequently, environmentalists in the United States—not the FDA—discovered that the unapproved Star Link corn had contaminated the food supply. More than three hundred products in grocery stores across the country were recalled. The costs of compensating farmers, grain buyers, food companies, and consumers from Star Link losses were estimated at nearly $1 billion.

According to a government document obtained by the Freedom of Information Act by the Center for Food Safety, the EPA and Bayer CropScience (then Aventis) knew that the corn entered the human food supply more than half a year before environmental advocates discovered it in taco shells[45] and brought it to the public's attention for a recall.

Bayer now sells Aventis' former biotech crops under the brand name Liberty Link (corn, soybeans, and canola). Liberty Link crops are genetically altered to tolerate high doses of the company's toxic herbicide glufosinate called Liberty.

Bayer is currently trying to commercialize its Liberty Link rice in the United States; rice is the number-one staple food in the world.[46] The director of the Louisiana State University AgCenter for Rice Research, Steve Linscombe, grew GE rice in field trials between 2001 and 2003, yet he didn't know how one of the GE rice lines, Bayer's Liberty Link long-grain rice, made its way into the food supply. When the contamination was announced in August 2006, Liberty Link had not been approved for human consumption; yet, within three months, the USDA deregulated the crop, retroactively claiming it was safe. Disavowing any responsibility, Bayer put the blame of contamination on farmers and said it was also an "act of God."[47]

Patent Applications

In light of Bayer's involvement in areas that affect the food supply, it is worth noting that in 2003, Bayer filed fifty-eight patent applications for new agrochemical substances, nearly twice as many patent applications as were filed by the two next-placed competitors combined. Bayer AG Management Board Chairman Werner Wenning, speaking at an investor conference in France, had high praise for Bayer CropScience's research activities: "We are convinced that Bayer is capable of sustained growth and high profitability, and that it can secure a competitive advantage through innovation ..."[48]

Failure to Disclose Fatal Consequences

With revenues of $35.5 billion in 2005, Bayer agreed to pay $8 million to settle a legal action by thirty states over its failure to disclose "sometimes fatal" consequences of using Baycol, a cholesterol-lowering drug. Bayer agreed that it failed to warn doctors and patients of the results of clinical studies that demonstrated "serious consequences" from using its drug.[49] This was another blatant example of how a company can do business at the expense of public health.

DuPont

DuPont was founded as a gunpowder maker in 1802 and has grown to be the world's largest chemical company. DuPont is also involved in synthetic fibers, electronics, and agricultural biotechnology.[50]

In the 1970s, DuPont was under scrutiny for its toxic products, such as leaded gasoline that damages the human nervous system and the chlorofluorocarbons (CFCs) in the refrigerant Freon that harm the ozone layer. At that time, top DuPont research executive Ed Jefferson read about and realized the commercial applications of genetic engineering. He invested in biotech for DuPont when he became chief executive officer in the early 1980s and even dedicated an $80 million DuPont lab to "life sciences."[51]

DuPont bought Pioneer Hi-Bred International in 1999, which made it the world's largest seed company. Pioneer was the largest company in the United States to use biotechnology to develop insect- or seed-resistant plants and produces corn, soy, alfalfa, canola, sorghum, sunflower, and wheat seeds. One of the leading producers of GE insect-resistant crops, Pioneer has also collaborated with Dow Chemical on an insect-resistant corn variety.[52] Pioneer owns dozens of seed-production facilities and more than one hundred research facilities worldwide.

Benomyl Exposure Birth Defects

In 2003, Florida judges awarded a family close to $7 million in damages from DuPont after their son had been born with empty eye sockets. It was the first time in history that a chemical company was found guilty of causing birth defects. "This is fantastic news; it shows that a large corporation cannot railroad over the terrible problems it has caused. My wife was exposed to Benlate very early-on in her pregnancy, and we are absolutely convinced that it caused our son's problems," the father commented.[53]

The safety of benomyl, the chemical ingredient of Benlate, had been questioned for years. As long ago as 1972, the EPA advised that DuPont should put a label on Benlate warning that it could "cause birth defects ... and exposure during pregnancy should be avoided."[54] But DuPont convinced the EPA that the warning would be misleading and unnecessary, so it never appeared.

An internal DuPont report about research that the company funded in 1997 by an independent laboratory in England during the legal dispute revealed that scientists had tested benomyl on rats and discovered that after two hours, a third of the benomyl was concentrated in the eyes, rising to two-thirds after twenty-four hours. After ten days, 80% of the benomyl was concentrated around the eyes.

DuPont disregarded the study and said humans could be exposed to large doses of the chemical without any risks to health. They denied that Benlate was the cause of the birth defects, saying the family's claim was based on "junk science."[55]

Concealed Teflon Dangers

In 1981, DuPont conducted a study to learn whether exposure to perfluorooctanoic acid (PFOA) caused birth defects in the children of Teflon factory workers. When the study resulted in an excess of birth defects in the children, it was hidden and DuPont did not notify the EPA. Under the Toxic Substances Control Act, companies must tell the EPA when they find information "that reasonably supports the conclusion that [a chemical] presents a substantial risk of injury to health."[56]

The EPA reported that exposure to even low levels of PFOA is harmful. More than fifty years after DuPont started producing Teflon near Parkersburg, West Virginia, federal officials accused the company of hiding information that suggested the chemical used to make Teflon causes cancer, birth defects, and other illnesses. "Someone made a conscious decision to expose us to this without telling us," said Robert Griffin, general manager of the Little Hocking Water Association, which supplies drinking water to twelve thousand customers from wells across the river that was contaminated with PFOA from the Teflon plant.[57]

For DuPont, revenues from biotechnology should exceed $1 billion over the next decade.[58]

REALITY CHECK

The truth about biotechnology has been subverted by "spin"—half-truths, omissions, and even exaggerations about results of growing GE food. Proponents of biotechnology continue to propagate myths about genetically altered crops, many of which have been proven to be untrue by the scientific community.

GE Crops Have Not Been Embraced Worldwide

Throughout the past decade, numerous national governments, just as in the United States, have invested heavily to build and expand research and development (R&D) capabilities and have implemented reforms to stimulate new biotech ventures and strategic partnerships. The biotech industry and governments would have the public believe that the world has embraced the technology.

Despite its growth, global GE crops remain limited. More than 80% of large-scale GE planting is limited to the United States, Argentina, and Canada, according to the Friends of the Earth International report *Who Benefits From GM Crops? Monsanto and Its Corporate-Driven Genetically Modified Revolution.* The one-hundred-dred-page analysis is about the global performance of GE crops from 1996 to 2006.[59]

The report concluded that:

- GE crops have led to an increase in herbicide use;

- GE crops do not address hunger and poverty issues; for instance, countries such as Indonesia and India have experienced substantial problems with GE crops, often leaving farmers heavily indebted;

- the biotech industry has failed to introduce GE crops with consumer benefits, and

- Monsanto has a formidable influence over governments and international bodies.

Notably, the increase in GE crops in a limited number of countries has been the result of the aggressive strategies of the biotech industry—not public acceptance.

Clive James, chairperson and founder of the industry-funded group International Service for the Acquisition of Agri-biotech Applications (ISAAA), has claimed an entire country to be accepting of GE crops—even if it grows just a single hectare. Claims made by James and the ISAAA have been challenged by opposing groups, which have questioned the ISAAA's claims on the acceptance of GE crops around the world and the benefits gained by producers. Greenpeace International reports have shown that resistance to GE crops continues to grow among farmers, consumers, and governments.

It is not known where ISAAA gets its data because the organization offers no references. James contends that ISAAA data is proprietary and is based on government and industry information. Even so, ISAAA statistics are widely quoted by governments and scientists. "If [Friends of the Earth International] reports had no references we'd be a laughing stock and yet ISAAA stats are widely quoted by governments and scientists," said Adrian Bebb of Friends of the Earth Europe.[60]

GE Crops Do Not Save Money and the Environment

In the 2002 study *Seeds of Doubt: North American Farmers' Experiences of GM Crops* conducted by the British Soil Association, the UK's leading campaigning and certification organization for organic food and farming, it was estimated that North America lost more than $12 billion due to GE food in the period from 1994 to 2000.[61] The study further revealed that:

- the profitability for farmers growing GE herbicide-tolerant soy and insect-resistant corn is less than non-GE crops;

- the lost export trade as a result of GE crops is thought to have caused a fall in farm prices, and hence, a need for increased government (taxpayer) subsidies—estimated at an extra $3-5 billion annually;

- the U.S. government has admitted that GE crops do not increase yields due to substantially reduced harvests;

- GE herbicide-resistance plants grow and spread quickly, causing farmers to spray with more herbicides, sometimes reverting to older, more toxic chemicals; and

- contamination of non-GE crops by GE crops is inevitable.

One challenge facing farmers today is that repeated use of glyphosate weed killer (Monsanto's Roundup) creates glyphosate-resistant weeds. In 2006, U.S. scientists discovered that giant ragweeds, or "superweeds," in Indiana and Ohio have become immune to glyphosate. In the southern United States where GE cotton is widely grown, 39% of farmers who grow GE crops reported problems with glyphosate-resistant weeds.[62] Just a few years ago, "superweeds" were non-existent.

GE Crops Do Not Feed the World

Biotech corporations, along with the U.S. government, claim that biotechnology is needed to feed the growing world population. Claiming an altruistic motivation for forcing biotechnology into the food supply is an easy way to garner support.

The reality is that several food security problems exist, and they will not be solved with GE food. In third-world countries, people are so poor that they cannot afford what is already grown. In fact, more than enough food is already being produced to provide the world with a nutritious and adequate diet—more than one-and-a-half times the amount required, according to the United Nations World Food Programme.[63] If people go hungry, it is not because of a shortage of food, but because complex social, political, and economic forces affect how people have access to land, money, and resources. There is more than enough food to feed everyone, yet more than 840 million people worldwide go hungry daily, and nearly two billion people are malnourished.[64]

In fact, most GE crops are destined for markets in wealthy countries. The majority of soy and corn is used for animal feed and for adding to processed food, which does not help feed the poor and hungry of the world.

Another problem is that industrial agricultural farms can produce food cheaper than what the poorest farmers of the third world can produce. When cheap food is sold or given to the third-world countries, it undermines and destroys local farm economies.

With a Ph.D. in political economics, Dr. J.W. Smith has written about the causes and cures of world poverty and has lectured at conferences around the world. In *World's Wasted Wealth 2*, he contends that if third-world farmers were given access to land, access to industrial tools, and were protected from cheap imports, they could become self-sufficient in food production. Reclaiming their land and utilizing unemployed citizens would cost these societies almost nothing, feed them well, and save far more money than they now pay for the so-called "cheap" imported foods.[65]

Steve Smith, an employee of biotech-giant Syngenta in 2003, asserted, "If anyone tells you that GM is going to feed the world, tell them that it is not ... To feed the world takes political and financial will. It's not about production and distribution."[66]

In June 1998, delegates from eighteen African countries at a meeting of the United Nations Food and Agriculture Organization responded to Monsanto's advertisements (with images of starving African children and how biotechnology is the solution to feeding the world's hungry) with the comment:

> We ... strongly object that the image of the poor and hungry from our countries is being used by giant multinational corporations to push a technology that is neither safe, environmentally friendly, nor economically beneficial to us. We do not believe that such companies or gene technologies will help our farmers to produce the food that is needed ... on the contrary ... it will undermine our capacity to feed ourselves.[67]
>
> What is being presented as an act of charity is in fact nothing more than an act of marketing.[68]

A group of academic researchers from South Africa, Mexico, and America claimed Monsanto has affected public opinion to reduce critical scrutiny, following tried-and-true public relations tactics. "The largest producer of commercial GM seeds, Monsanto, exemplifies the industry's strategies: the invocation of poor people as beneficiaries, characterization of opposition as technophobic or anti-progress, and portrayal of their products as environmentally beneficial in the absence of or despite the evidence ... This [public relations] strategy removes debate that is vital for public and environmental health, particularly when the risks and benefits of GM crops still remain undecided at best ..."[69]

When the U.S. government and the biotech industry assert that mass production of GE foods is necessary to feed the world, how is it possible that 11% of the population in the United States lacked food in 2005? According to Economic Research Service's report *Household Food Security in the United States, 2005*, there has been a continuing trend in growing hunger in the United States over the past five years.[70]

Following the logic of the biotech industry and the U.S. government (that hunger is caused solely by a shortage of food), how is it possible that people in the United States go hungry—at a time when U.S. acreage of GE crops is enormous and growing? When has biotech food *ever* contributed to solving hunger?

GE Crops Rarely Produce Higher Yields

Research has shown that the agricultural performance of biotech crops is worse than conventional varieties. So why are millions of acres of GE crops being grown?

The Economic Research Service released an analysis of the economic performance of GE crops in America, using USDA survey data to examine the extent to which U.S. farmers have adopted bioengineered crops, factors affecting adoption of these crops, and the impacts of bioengineered crops on usage and net returns. The 2002 report *The Adoption of Bioengineered Crops* revealed that most of the basic economic claims made for GE crops are either false or questionable, and that "perhaps the biggest issue raised by these results is how to explain the rapid adoption of GE crops when farm financial impacts appear to be mixed or even negative."[71]

The British Soil Association's 2002 report *Seeds of Doubt* determined that the main reason farmers have said they choose GE crops is for increased yields. However, on average, the claims of increased yield have not been realized for most GE crops and some have reduced yields, such as Roundup soy and canola. Yet, the myth of economic benefits continues to be propagated by those with vested interests. Missouri farmer and president of the U.S. Family Farm Coalition, Bill Christison, said at a conference on Biodevastation in 1998, "The promise was that you could use less chemicals and produce greater yield. But let me tell you none of this is true."[72]

Dr. Charles Hagedorn, professor of Crop and Soil Environmental Sciences at Virginia Tech University, is an extension specialist working with Virginia State University and the USDA. An extension specialist is responsible for communicating unbiased, independent research findings to farmers, giving them access to proven scientific research when selecting crop varieties. However, the extension specialists are being circumvented, and farmers are now sold GE seeds directly from biotech representatives. According to Dr. Hagedorn,

> Now, the Ag [agricultural biotech] companies are going directly to the farmers with contracts for growing their GM crops, and the extension crop specialist is 'out of the loop.' In the U.S., sales of the GM crops to farmers have gone wild ... This is a classic case of what has been described in the literature as a situa-

tion where commercial development and marketing is way ahead of the science.[73]

GE Crops Are Not Rigorously Regulated

One would hope that the U.S. government would do everything possible to ensure that GE food is safe for consumers and the environment; however, in the case of biotechnology, the U.S. government seems to act more on behalf of wealthy special interests than for the public it is supposed to serve.

In June 2005, Charles Lambert, deputy under secretary of agriculture for regulatory programs at the U.S. State Department, claimed that the three U.S. agencies responsible for regulating agricultural biotechnology (USDA, FDA, and EPA) "are working to assure industry, consumers, and other groups both in the United States and abroad that genetically engineered crops, animal vaccines, and other products are rigorously regulated for safety."[74] Addressing the Senate Agriculture Committee, he stressed the importance of public confidence in government regulation.

Unfortunately for consumers, not only are GE foods *not* safety tested, but they are also *not* rigorously regulated.

The USDA has the responsibility of overseeing GE crops. Companies that want to commercialize crops must petition the USDA, but the USDA has not established rigorous rules to prevent GE crops from contaminating conventional crops. The USDA permits cultivation of GE pharmaceutical crops, despite contamination incidents with corn and soybeans, and they do not test neighboring fields for GE contamination.[75]

In a report released in December 2005, the inspector general of the USDA criticized many aspects of the oversight of GE crops and charged that the branch of the USDA that oversees biotechnology regulatory functions was not complying with the regulations it was supposed to be following regarding field-trial monitoring of biotech crops.

In February 2007, a federal judge ruled that the USDA violated the law by neglecting to assess possible environmental impacts before approving Monsanto's

GE alfalfa. Alfalfa is the fourth most widely planted crop in the United States—a huge market for Monsanto to penetrate.

Judge Charles R. Breyer of Federal District Court in San Francisco said the USDA had been "cavalier" in deciding that a full environmental impact statement was not needed because the potential environmental and economic effects of the crop were not significant. He said that the agency had not considered the possibility that the gene could be transferred by pollen to organic or conventional alfalfa, hurting sales of organic farmers or exports to countries like Japan that did not want the GE variety. He commented, "An action which potentially eliminates or at least greatly reduces the availability of a particular plant, here, non-engineered alfalfa, has a significant effect on the human environment."[76]

The EPA has the responsibility for licensing pesticides and regulating pesticide-producing GE plants. Genetically altered Bt plants, which include corn, cotton, and potatoes, synthesize their own bacterial protein to kill pests. When the EPA allowed Bt corn on the market, the agency only reviewed the studies provided by biotech companies that stood to benefit financially.

For its part, the FDA is responsible for protecting the public health by assuring, among other things, the safety of our nation's food supply.

When determining the regulation of GE food, the FDA has relied on the Food, Drug, and Cosmetic Act (FD&C Act), originally passed in 1938. In essence, the FD&C Act requires the pre-market approval of *food additives* intentionally added to food; otherwise, foods bypass pre-market approval if they are considered to be Generally Recognized As Safe (GRAS).[77] A GRAS substance is distinguished from a food additive based on the common knowledge about the safety of the substance for its intended use. The FD&C Act was written—long before GE food entered our food supply—to address the growing number of chemical additives used in food. It was not intended to regulate modern agricultural biotechnology.

Because the FDA asserted that GE crops are "substantially equivalent" to conventional, non-GE crops in the 1992 *Statement of Food Policy*, based on the fact that nothing was "added" to the final food product, the same regulation applies to bioengineered foods as to their conventional counterparts. Therefore, GE whole foods such as fruits, vegetables, and grains are not subject to pre-market approval because "they have been used for food for lengthy periods of time and are presumed to be GRAS."[78] The FDA's key factor in assessing GE food safety relates to the characteristics of the food product, *not the method used to produce the product.*

As James Maryanski, FDA's biotechnology coordinator in 1999, put it: "Because FDA determined that bioengineered foods should be regulated like their conventional counterparts, FDA has not to date established any regulations specific to bioengineered food."[79]

Michael Pollan's article *Playing God in the Garden,* published in *The New York Times* in October 1998, exemplified the lack of regulation of biotech food in the United States in the case of Monsanto's GE "New Leaf" potato.

Introduced in 1995, the New Leaf Bt potato was registered with the EPA as a pesticide, poisonous to the Colorado copper beetle. The FDA is responsible for food labeling but does not have the authority to label pesticides; that responsibility falls on the EPA. The labels on Monsanto's GE potatoes listed the nutrients in the potatoes, but there was no reference that the potatoes were genetically altered to produce a pesticide in every one of its cells.

EPA-approved pesticides have warning labels, including Bt pesticides. However, because the Monsanto Bt potato was food, the EPA said the FDA was responsible for labeling. But the FDA can't include any information about pesticides on its food labels; therefore, the FDA did not regulate Monsanto's potato, because the FDA does not have the authority to regulate pesticides. That is the EPA's responsibility.

Pollan also stated that for other food crops that are not Bt or registered pesticides, the FDA has the authority to regulate them. Since 1992, however, they have allowed companies like Monsanto to decide for themselves if their products are safe, thus avoiding regulation.[80]

The FDA has been under fire for lack of food safety and oversight. As a result, in May 2007, the agency created the new post of "Food Safety Czar." The FDA named Dr. David Acheson, chief medical officer at the FDA's Center for Food Safety and Applied Nutrition, as assistant commissioner for food protection, who will also be the FDA's liaison with the U.S. Health and Human Services Department, the USDA, and other federal agencies involved in food safety issues. Representative Rosa DeLauro, a senior member of the House Appropriations Committee, criticized the FDA by saying, "The agency should already have a sense of the barriers, gaps, and most critical needs in our food safety system."[81]

Former FDA commissioner David Kessler told the House Oversight and Government Reform Committee at a congressional hearing, "The food safety system in this country is broken. Food safety can't be delegated to second-tier management within the agency, and the fact is that food is a second-tier priority within the FDA."[82]

Contrary to what the government would have the public believe, regulatory agencies are not rigorously regulating the food supply. Questions, contradictions, and doubts surrounding the appropriate regulation and safety of GE foods are widespread.

A peer-reviewed scientific study, *Safety Testing and Regulation of Genetically Engineered Foods*, published in 2004 in *Biotechnology and Genetic Engineering Reviews*, affirmed that GE crops are not thoroughly tested, not regulated, nor are they proven safe. The report revealed flaws both in the way biotech companies test and in the way the U.S. government regulates GE crops. It included a case study of two types of insecticide-producing Bt corn, but focused on Monsanto's MON810 Bt corn.[83] Authors Dr. David Schubert, cell biologist and medical researcher at California's Salk Institute, and William Freese, research analyst with Friends of the Earth U.S., based their report on approximately one hundred sources, including U.S. regulatory documents and unpublished studies by biotech companies.

Schubert and Freese found many biotech testing flaws, such as the use of substitute GE proteins for testing rather than the GE plant-produced proteins that people actually consume; the failure of companies to test for unintended effects of the unpredictable GE process; the lack of long-term animal-feeding studies; and the way biotech companies manipulate tests to get desired results.

"One thing that surprised us is that U.S. regulators rely almost exclusively on information provided by the biotech crop developer, and those data are not published in journals or subjected to peer review," said Schubert. "The picture that emerges from our study of U.S. regulation of GM foods is a rubber-stamp approval process designed to increase public confidence in, but not ensure the safety of, genetically engineered foods."[84]

Overall, U.S. regulatory agencies' policies state that: no public records need to be kept on farms growing GE crops; companies that buy from farmers and sell to food manufacturers and grocery chains do not need to keep GE crops separate from traditional crops (therefore purchasers have no way to avoid buying GE foods); and labeling of any seeds, crops, or any food products with information about their GE origins is not required.[85] *As a result of these policies, American consumers have no way to exercise informed choices in the grocery store.*

RISKY BUSINESS

"How do commercial interests usually protect themselves from liability claims?" Dr. David Suzuki asked. "Through insurance. In fact, the litmus test for safety is insurance. You can be insured for almost anything if you pay enough for the premium, but if the insurance industry isn't willing to bet its money on the safety of a product or technology, it means the risks are simply too high or too uncertain for them to take the gamble."[86]

The European community expressed some concerns over the safety of GE foods in 1999. London's newspaper *The Independent* declared:

> European governments have drawn up contingency plans for a nuclear fallout-style emergency involving genetically modified organisms. A five-point Emergency Response Plan has been formulated by the European Commission, designed to cope if genetically modified plants result in widespread illness or the death of wildlife ... The plan is designed to prevent a human health disaster and stop genetically modified plants from breeding wildly with native species.[87]

No insurance company has ever been willing to insure the biotech industry. GE crops, like war and nuclear accidents, have been deemed too dangerous to insure.[88] Insurance companies do not provide farmers, their neighbors, or anyone else coverage against the risks of GE contamination. In short, if insurance companies conclude that GE crops are unsafe, how can the American public be expected to believe that the food they eat every day is safe?

Chapter 2
Science Under the Influence

There is a profound difference between the types of unexpected effects from traditional breeding and genetic engineering ... There is no certainty that the breeders of GM foods will be able to pick up effects that might not be obvious.

This is the industry's pet idea, namely that there are no unintended effects that will raise the FDA's level of concern. But time and time again, there is no data to back up their contention.[1]
Dr. Louis Pribyl of the FDA microbiology group in a March 1992 memo to FDA's biotechnology coordinator James Maryanski

We are told there is rigorous testing, but where is it? It is not published in any of the journals. The politicians have been saying this bit of nonsense that GM foods are the most rigorously tested food in the history of mankind ... The truth is different, however.

You can count the number of relevant peer-reviewed papers on the fingers of your hands. I have a feeling that any unbiased observer would say that this is a very poor record for an industry that is just about to save the world from famine and other calamities.[2]
Scientist Dr. Arpad Pusztai, quoted in Sheldon Rampton's and John Stauber's Trust Us, We're Experts

The biotech industry often refers to people opposed to GE food as anti-science, irrational, anti-technology, uninformed, and emotional. On the contrary, biotech critics have legitimate concerns and want more science to gain a science-based, rational policy on GE food.

GE food poses real risks. What is lacking is scientific proof of its safety.

CONFLICTS OF INTEREST

Science in the public interest in the United States has led to scientific progress and leadership in the global community. However, the collaboration between public and private sectors has compromised science considerably. In particular, agricultural research and development (R&D) has been significantly influenced by the consolidation of chemical, seed, and biotechnology companies.

Corporate-funded science is a problem when there are conflicts of interest between a company's marketing agenda and the public's right to know about possible adverse health or environmental risks. When research results are not to a sponsor's liking, a company can suppress undesirable research results, even if it risks public health.[3] The *London Telegraph* article *Scientists Asked to Fix Results for Backer* explained that contracting out and the commercialization of scientific research are threatening standards of impartiality. The article quoted Dr. Richard Smith, former editor of *British Medical Journal*, who said competing interests that sponsor research have "quite a profound influence on the conclusions and we deceive ourselves if we think science is wholly impartial."[4]

The Funding Effect

Before 1980, collaboration between public and private sectors was limited because the private sector could not claim ownership of inventions or patents that resulted from federally funded research. Federal researchers had not been allowed to work directly with the private sector, but that changed when the 1980 Bayh-Dole Act granted all institutions "certainty of title" for inventions or patents resulting from federally funded research.

In addition, the 1986 Technology Transfer Act allowed government agencies to convert federally funded scientific findings into profitable private-sector products. It authorized federal agencies to enter into R&D agreements with other federal agencies, public and private foundations, and nonprofit organizations, including universities; it also permits employees or former employees of the laboratory to participate in efforts to commercialize inventions they made while in the public sector.[5]

University faculty members involved in corporate-sponsored biotech research are often vested in the same companies in which they do research, while being paid as consultants or advisory committees, and they often benefit financially.[6] "Virtually every academic in biotechnology is involved in exploiting [science] commercially," the late Orville Chapman, professor of chemistry and biochemistry at the University of California at Los Angeles, commented in 2002. "We've lost our credentials as unbiased on such subjects as cloning or the modification of living things, and we seem singularly reluctant to think it through."[7]

Economic interests, rather than science, have been the motivation for the change in government policy. The timing of the passage of the Bayh-Dole Act and the Technology Transfer Act could not have been better for the biotech industry. The acts were passed within a few years of when the U.S. Supreme Court and the U.S. Patent and Trademark Office issued a ruling that all GE living organisms are patentable. Private-sector agricultural R&D has increased, which has been driven by advances in biotechnology, increased patent rights, and new opportunities to collaborate with public research institutions.

One example was an agreement between Novartis (now Syngenta) and the University of California at Berkeley.[8] Syngenta gave Berkeley $25 million for research in agricultural biotechnology, which in turn allowed Syngenta access to DNA databases and proprietary technology. The university owns the patents and earns royalties from any discoveries made during the contract, and in return, Syngenta has the first rights to license about 30-40% of any biotech "inventions."

The University of Nebraska at Lincoln partnered with Monsanto in March 2005. Researchers are to receive up to $2.5 million from Monsanto between 2005 and 2010 to develop soybean seeds that can withstand sprayings of a particular weed killer. The agreement also calls for royalty payments to the university after the seed goes to market. University of Nebraska Regent Chuck Hassebrook, executive director of the Center for Rural Affairs, a nonprofit organization that advocates for small family farms, criticized the agreement, claiming that the university's research is helping Monsanto get richer, and said, "What we're doing is going to suck money out of rural Nebraska and put it into the corporate coffers in St. Louis ... Monsanto makes more money, and farmers make less."[9]

Dr. Sheldon Krimsky, professor of urban and environmental policy and planning, School of Arts and Sciences at Tufts University and adjunct professor in the Department of Public Health and Family Medicine at the Tufts School of Medicine in Massachusetts, also pointed out, "Today, biotechnology and pharmaceutical companies regularly give universities multi-million-dollar grants ... At the same time, universities and their professors are plunging into the business world themselves, creating companies to sell products discovered in academic laboratories."[10] Dr. Krimsky calls it "the funding effect in science," in which research results favor the financial interests of their sponsors.

In his book *Science in the Private Interest*, he contends that the funding effect has arrived at universities, and as a result, they are no longer independent sources of reliable, objective information. One might believe there are oversights, such as federal advisory boards. But Dr. Krimsky said, "There are two rules that guide federal advisory committees: Rule number one is that no scientist with a substantial conflict of interest should be permitted to serve on an advisory committee. Rule number two is that rule number one can be waived. And the number of waivers is extraordinary."[11]

A study Dr. Krimsky conducted in the late 1980s found that 37% of the biotechnology scientists who were members of the National Academy of Sciences, an organization that advises Congress and the federal government on science policy, had "industry affiliations," making their decisions on biotech science policies questionable.[12] He concluded that commercially driven biotech research has negatively affected the sharing of ideas and has slowed cooperative efforts to find solutions to problems, because academic scientists are under pressure to find commercial uses for their research so that their institution can patent, license, and profit from the work.

In 1994 and 1995, researchers led by Dr. David Blumenthal, director of the Institute for Health Policy at Massachusetts General Hospital, surveyed more than 3,000 academic researchers involved in "life sciences" and found that 64% of the scientists reported having a financial relationship with private industry.

They also found that scientists with industry relationships were more likely to delay or withhold publication of their data if it produced undesirable results for the sponsor. Their study, published by the *Journal of the American Medical Association*,[13] found that the practice of withholding publication or refusing to share data with other scientists was common among biotechnology researchers.

Scientists Censored

As corporate influence continues to rise, so does the suppression of scientific dissent. Dr. David Suzuki commented in *Biotechnology: A Geneticist's Perspective*,

> Students are presented with one-sided information about the potential benefits of these areas with little balance from those with concerns ... In my experience, merely questioning the activity or suggesting possible hazards is to invite strong disapproval and accusation of being "anti-science" or "emotional and non-scientific." It is a sad state in a so-called community of scholars where dissent or difference of opinions is supposed to be valued.[14]

One example is the case of well-respected microbial biologist and professor at the University of California (UC) at Berkeley, Dr. Ignacio Chapela, who was fired after publishing a scientific report regarding the uncontrolled contamination of native Mexican corn varieties by GE corn. An important fact is that biotech corporation Novartis, now Syngenta, provided the university $50 million in funding over a five-year period beginning in 1998.

Chapela was concerned that corn in Mexico was being inundated by cheap biotech U.S. and Canadian corn after the passage of the North American Free Trade Agreement. As a member of the National Academy of Science's committee reviewing the impacts of GE crops, Dr. Chapela had raised questions about contamination of non-GE crops with GE varieties, particularly from U.S.-exported agriculture.

In 2000, Dr. Chapela sent graduate student David Quist to Oaxaca, Mexico to investigate the contamination of the native, heirloom corn by GE corn. Quist returned to Berkeley with samples and the results were confirmed in March 2001. When an article Chapela and Quist wrote for the British scientific journal *Nature* describing their discovery was published in November 2001, Dr. Chapela's academic career would be in jeopardy.

According to the article *The Sad Saga of Ignacio Chapela* by John Ross,

> Big Biotech, alerted to the Mexican corn study in advance sought to preempt publication by hiring a high-powered Washington PR firm, the Bivings Group, which specializes in internet subterfuge. The Chapela-Quist study had barely touched down on the newsstands when an orchestrated barrage of letters decried "fundamental flaws" in the research ... Investigative reportage by the British *Guardian* failed to verify the existence of the authors, but traced the computer used to generate the e-mail campaign to one operated by a Bivings front.[15]

In November 2003, Chapela was denied tenure, even though a review panel had previously voted to approve him.

Chapela filed a lawsuit against the university, claiming that they had made an example out of him and that UC removed him due to pressure from Novartis [Syngenta]. "The university has lost the capacity to do science ... This is not a lawsuit against the university; it is a lawsuit for the university and against the people who have bastardized and taken away what the university used to do."[16] He further commented, "I am living proof of what happens when biotech buys a university. The first thing that goes is independent research. The university is a delicate organism. When its mission and orientation are compromised, it dies. Corporate biotechnology is killing this university."[17]

In May 2005, after personal hardship, media attention, and public protests on his behalf, the university finally granted tenure to Chapela.

Another example of suppression occurred with scientist Dr. Arpad Pusztai. Throughout his nearly fifty-year career, Dr. Pusztai worked at universities and research institutes in Budapest, London, Chicago, and Scotland. It was in Scotland where he worked at the Rowett Research Institute for thirty-five years. He had published approximately three hundred primary peer-reviewed papers and wrote or edited twelve scientific books. He led research about the effects of dietary lectins on the gastrointestinal tract, including those in GE crop plants.

When Dr. Pusztai and his team began researching GE foods in the UK in 1995, they searched for biological tests that had been conducted on GE foods and found none—even though, at that time, GE food had been consumed by the public for more than a year. But the following year in 1996, Dr. Pusztai found a study published in the *Journal of Nutrition* written by B.G. Hammond, a Monsanto scientist.[18] After feeding Monsanto's GE Roundup Ready soybeans to rats, catfish, chickens, and cows, Hammond concluded that the GE soy had the same nutritional value as conventional soybeans.[19]

Dr. Pusztai thought Hammond's paper lacked validity: "Monsanto used mature animals that do not form body tissues and organs; adults only need a small amount of protein because their bodies are in equilibrium, but a young growing animal needs a great deal more protein because it's laying down muscle and tissues and forming its organs." Also important is the fact that there was only a small amount, about 7%, of GE soy in their diet. He further commented, "It was obvious that the study had been designed to avoid finding any problems ..."[20]

At the time, Dr. Pusztai still considered himself a supporter of biotechnology, so he began his own feeding experiments with rats and expected there to be no problems with the GE potatoes he was testing.[21] However, the rats fed on GE potatoes showed unexpected changes in the size and weight of their body organs, including smaller livers, hearts, and brains, and his research team also found evidence of weakened immune systems.[22]

Dr. Pusztai warned the UK Ministry of Agriculture about his concerns, and in 1998, he warned government inspectors. He said in a British Broadcasting Corporation (BBC) interview that the potatoes caused weakened immune systems: "If it is left to me, I will certainly not eat it. We are putting new things into food that have not been eaten before. The effects on the immune system are not predictable, and I challenge anyone who will say that the effects are predictable."[23]

After going public in that BBC interview with the results of his potato study, Dr. Pusztai was fired from the Rowett Research Institute and threatened with a lawsuit. (According to Joel Bleifuss in his 2000 article *No Small Genetic Potatoes* in *In These Times*, the Rowett Institute received a $224,000 grant from Monsanto prior to Pusztai's BBC interview and firing.) In February 1999, twenty-two scientists from thirteen countries signed a public statement in support of Dr. Pusztai, expressing concern over the attack on scientific freedom. Following extensive review and debate, he was exonerated but was not allowed to continue his important research. Even so, his study was published in *The Lancet* in October that same year.[24]

Eight years later in 2007, campaigners against GE crops in Britain demanded trials of GE potatoes to be stopped after more evidence of links with cancers in laboratory rats had been released to the public. In particular, Irina Ermakova, a Russian scientist and consultant for Greenpeace, said, "The GM potatoes were the most dangerous of the feeds used in the trials ... and on the basis of this evidence, they cannot be used in the nourishment of people." UK Greenpeace activists said the Russian findings, after an eight-year court battle with the biotech industry, vindicated Pusztai's research.[25] Alan Simpson, a Labour Member of Parliament and activist, said, "These trials should be stopped. The research backs up the work of Arpad Pusztai, and it shows that he was the victim of a smear campaign by the biotech industry. There has been a cover up over these findings and the government should not be a party to that."[26]

Peer-Reviewed Journals

Motivated by the awareness of increasing academic-industry collaborations and of scientists who author research with financial ties to favorable results, scientific journals introduced conflict of interest (COI) policies in the 1980s.

Dr. Sheldon Krimsky conducted a study in 1996 that looked into industry connections of the authors of 789 scientific papers published by 1,105 researchers in fourteen life science and biomedical journals. In 34% of the papers, at least one of the head authors had a financial interest connected to the research. It was concluded that the estimate of 34% was probably lower than the true level of financial COI because he was unable to check if the researchers owned stock or had received consulting fees from the companies involved in commercial applications of their research. None of the financial interests were disclosed in the journals where readers could identify them.[27]

The following year, Dr. Krimsky conducted a study, which revealed that only 16% of 1,396 biomedical journals had COI policies and less than 1% of the articles published during that year in the journals with COI policies contained any disclosures of the authors' personal financial interests.[28]

An example of conflict of interest was exposed in the press release *Journal Editors Urged to Disclose Conflicts of Interest* by the Center for Science in the Public Interest in 2003. Scientist Roger Beachy, director of Missouri's Danforth Plant

Science Center, a research institute dedicated to plant biotechnology research, published an editorial on the safety of GE crops in *Science* magazine and cosigned a letter in *Nature Biotechnology*. Neither journal disclosed that Beachy's research on agricultural biotechnology had been funded by Monsanto and other biotech companies, even though he had written about the safety of GE crops, which was directly relevant to those companies.[29]

As academic research dollars flow from corporate sponsors, conflicts of interest in the biotech industry are undermining and distorting real science. As Dr. Krimsky put it: "The term 'conflict of interest' is like a flashing yellow signal to alert society to proceed with caution in the face of some actual or potential wrongdoing, or bias, primarily among people who hold positions of public trust … COI disclosure is relevant to reviewers of articles because it provides them with a skepticism that they need to give a good review. Skepticism is good for science. Reviewers need to come to articles with some skepticism."[30]

Confidential Business Information

Much industry research on biotech food is not reported in peer-reviewed literature where it can be scientifically reviewed. In fact, it can be kept out of public domain if a company claims a report contains "confidential business information."

In 2002, Monsanto's MON863 corn, a genetically altered Bt corn that produces its own pesticide designed to be resistant to the root worm in each one of its cells, was approved in the United States. *As far as U.S. regulatory agencies are concerned, if Monsanto says its products are safe, that is enough for approval; at the same time, Monsanto retains the right not to release information in the United States about their products based on "confidential business information."*

In 2005, Monsanto tried to get Europe's approval for MON863, but Monsanto maintained that research on the corn contained confidential business information and should not be available for public view.

Greenpeace International in Germany wanted access to the research document because of a law in the European Union that says the public has the right to see all documents related to risk assessments of GE plants. After German authorities gave Greenpeace access, Monsanto filed a court case against the German government to stop publication. However, the German court ordered Monsanto to make their ninety-day-rat study public in June 2005.[31]

The study revealed many *statistically significant* differences with the rats fed MON863 corn. The rats developed adverse reactions, including those typically found in response to allergies, infections, toxins, and various diseases including cancer. The reactions were also those that are typical in the presence of anemia and blood pressure problems. In addition, there were increased blood sugar levels, liver and kidney lesions, kidney inflammation, and other changes. Even though rats fed Monsanto's GE corn had serious health problems, Monsanto scientists concluded that the health problems were irrelevant and should not be attributed to the GE corn itself, even though the rats fed non-GE did not have those problems. [32, 33]

According to Dr. Arpad Pusztai, who was commissioned by the German government to evaluate the study, "What is the point of doing a study if you dismiss the results you find? It is almost impossible to imagine that major lesions in important organs ... or changes in blood parameters ... that occurred in GM maize-fed rats, is incidental and due to simple biological variability," as Monsanto claimed.[34]

French professor Gilles Eric Seralini, a French government scientist and expert in GE technology from the University of Caen, said that the results indicated a toxic reaction. Seralini is a member of two French government commissions that evaluate GE food; one of those commissions originally rejected a request for approval of MON863 in October 2003 due to the adverse results of the study. However, Seralini was told by French authorities in 2003 that he was legally bound to keep his opinions confidential.[35]

Only because of the Greenpeace International lawsuit in Germany were Seralini and Pusztai finally given the opportunity to expose Monsanto's flawed study in June 2005. Until then, however, Monsanto had been able to keep their feeding study hidden for two years by claiming that confidential business information was in the report. Even so, MON863 corn was approved for human consumption in the United States in 2006. It is deplorable that the FDA believes U.S. consumers should not be permitted to know which foods contain GE ingredients and which do not.

THE EMPEROR'S (FDA'S) BIOTECH CLOTHES

You might assume, or at least, hope, that the U.S. government would do every-thing to ensure that GE foods are safe for American consumers and the environ-ment. Even FDA scientists, among other scientists, have expressed concerns over the safety of GE foods, which have never been proven safe through independent scientific testing. The belief that they are safe stems from an unfounded assump-tion, propagated by the FDA and the biotech industry.

FDA Sued by Its Own Scientists

In 1998, nine eminent scientists, including some of the FDA's own scientists, biologists, and advisers, sued the FDA to require mandatory safety testing and labeling of GE foods. Along with public interest attorney and director of the Alli-ance for Bio-Integrity Steven Drucker, they formed a coalition and were joined by consumer groups, religious organizations, and other concerned scientists, who claimed that every GE food in the United States is on the market illegally and should be recalled for rigorous safety testing.[36] Contradicting the FDA's own claims that its 1992 *Statement of Food Policy* is science-based and bioengineered foods are GRAS by the scientific community, files proved that agency scientists warned the FDA that biotech foods are riskier than conventionally produced foods and that the FDA ignored those warnings.[37]

Dr. Louis Priybl of the FDA microbiology group wrote in a memo about the *Statement of Food Policy* in 1992 to James Maryanski, the FDA's biotechnology coordinator,

> What has happened to the scientific elements of this document? Without a sound scientific base to rest on, this becomes a broad, general, "What do I have to do to avoid trouble"-type document [for biotech companies]. A scien-tific document is needed ... It reads very pro-industry, especially in the area of unintended [health] effects, but contains very little input from consumers and only a few answers for their concerns ...

> There is a profound difference between the types of unexpected effects from traditional breeding and genetic engineering ... This is the industry's pet idea, namely that there are no unintended effects that will raise the FDA's level of concern. But time and time again, there is no data to back up their conten-tion.[38]

Linda Kahl, an FDA compliance officer, said, "The processes of genetic engineering and traditional breeding are different, and according to the technical experts at the agency, they lead to different risks." She also said the agency "was trying to fit a square peg into a round hole by trying to force an ultimate conclusion that there is no difference between foods modified and traditional."[39]

Likewise, Dr. Philip J. Regal, professor of ecology, behavior, and evolution at the University of Minnesota at St. Paul, commented,

> It is my considered judgment that the evidence to date ... indicates there are scientifically justified concerns about the safety of genetically engineered foods and that some of them could be quite dangerous ... Government scientist after scientist acknowledged there was no way to assure the safety of genetically engineered foods ... Several expressed the idea that, in order to take this important step of progress, society was going to have to bear an unavoidable measure of risk.[40]

The judge in this lawsuit, Coleen Kollar-Kotelly, acknowledged the FDA's files contained statements from its scientists warning about harmful side effects of GE foods and criticizing the lack of scientific basis for the FDA's policy. However, she said that the agency was legally entitled to establish policy, despite the contrary opinion of their own scientific staff.[41] The judge did *not* acknowledge that FDA administrators had not only disregarded the information from their scientists, but also denied they knew about it. The 1992 *Statement of Food Policy* states, "The agency is not aware of any information showing that foods derived by these new methods differ from other foods in any meaningful or uniform way."[42, 43]

The judge's final ruling upheld the FDA's policy on a technicality. The scientists' burden was to prove that FDA administrators had abused their discretion by acting arbitrarily and capriciously in adopting the presumption that GE foods are generally recognized as safe. *The issue was whether FDA administrators had acted arbitrarily and capriciously in presuming that GE foods are safe, not that GE foods are actually safe.*

Ultimately, the judge claimed that the 1992 *Statement of Food Policy* be upheld, even though she did not rule that GE foods have been generally recognized as safe among FDA scientists or within the scientific community.[44] The generally-recognized-as-safe claim is the legal basis for the U.S. marketing and non-labeling of GE foods, despite the fact that FDA officials know there is disagreement in the scientific community.

Another FDA Lawsuit

The Center for Food Safety (CFS) filed a lawsuit in June 2006 against the FDA to respond to the citizens' petition that CFS filed in March 2000 against the agency. The unanswered petition demanded mandatory reviews and labeling of GE foods.

The FDA's policy asserts that GE foods are safe based on the information that biotechnology companies voluntarily provide. Other countries have imposed mandatory pre-market approval and labeling systems for GE foods, including Russia, China, Brazil, India, Japan, Australia, New Zealand, South Korea, and the entire European Union.

For citizens in other countries, the FDA and other U.S. officials have endorsed three safety assessments and pre-market review agreements intended to protect consumers from the risks of GE foods. Those agreements are the Precautionary Principle, the Cartagena Protocol on Biosafety, and the Codex Alimentarius Commission's pre-market safety assessment documents. Even so, the FDA's guidelines for American consumers do not follow these same international safety standards.

The *Wingspread Statement on the Precautionary Principle* is a warning that was defined by more than eight hundred scientists from eighty-three countries about the hazards of and calling for a moratorium on all GE foods. It stated (in part): "… it is necessary to implement the Precautionary Principle when an activity raises threats of harm to human health or the environment; precautionary measures should be taken even if some cause and effect relationships are not fully established scientifically. In this context, the proponent of an activity, rather than the public, should bear the burden of proof of safety … The process of applying the Precautionary Principle must be open, informed, and democratic, and must include potentially affected parties …"[45]

The United Nations' Environmental Program's governing body of the Convention on Biological Diversity adopted an international agreement known as the Cartagena Protocol on Biosafety, seeking to protect biological diversity from the potential risks posed by living modified organisms (LMOs), or genetically modified organisms, resulting from modern biotechnology. The Protocol takes into consideration the precautionary approach and establishes an agreement procedure for ensuring that countries are provided with the documentation necessary to make informed decisions before agreeing to import LMOs/GMOs into their territory.

According to the United Nations' Environment Program's legal officer Worku Damena Yifru, "We believe the Protocol contributes to ensuring the safe movement and introduction of LMOs into the environment. In that regard, we feel that it is making a difference since its entry into force ... The Biosafety Protocol is not only based on the precautionary approach but also on a case-by-case risk assessment rule ... The Protocol has now 138 Parties. This is a significant trend for its future."[46]

The United States, the largest producer and promoter of biotech foods, is not a member.

The Codex Alimentarius Commission released its 2003 report *The Principles for the Risk Analysis of Foods Derived from Modern Biotechnology*, which provides a framework for evaluating the safety and nutritional aspects of GE foods. The commission is operated by the UN's Food and Agriculture Organization (FAO) and the World Health Organization (WHO). The Codex report says there is a need for a pre-market safety assessment of all GE foods on a case-by-case basis. The agreement is not legally binding but has been agreed to by all member nations.

According to FAO and WHO, the assessment addresses intended and unintended impacts of GE foods, identifying hazards and changes relevant to human health, especially regarding key nutrients and potential allergenic components.

In June 2005, WHO called for further safety assessments and a case-by-case risk assessment on GMOs, which should make governments more cautious before giving their approval for wider use of the technology. "Therefore, the potential human health effects of new GM foods should always be assessed before they are grown and marketed, and long-term monitoring must be carried out to catch any possible adverse effects early."[47]

Other governments take their role seriously in protecting public health and require precautionary measures; unfortunately, such protections do not apply to American consumers. Joe Mendelson, legal director of CFS, declared,

> While the rest of the world is rejecting these risky, untested foods, the FDA's unscientific approach is making American consumers the world's guinea pigs in this genetic food experiment. Americans deserve the right to know what's in their food. The FDA must stop playing politics and start developing a science-based policy to protect Americans from these risky foods.[48]

In August 2006, CFS "won" the lawsuit by forcing the FDA to answer their six-year-old petition; however, the FDA denied CFS's efforts and any further responsibility to the American public regarding the testing or labeling of GE foods.

The Department of Health and Human Service's assistant commissioner for policy, Jeffrey Shuren, responded on behalf of the FDA to CFS's petition. He maintained that transferred genetic material does not raise a safety concern as a component of food, that GE food is presumed to be generally recognized as safe, and said that the key factor in assessing safety relates to the characteristics of the food product, not the method used to produce the product.

Shuren commented that the FDA believes consumers' desire for labeling is not important: "… consumer interest alone is not a sufficient government interest in which to compel labeling" and that testing is unnecessary to determine adverse health effects: "… you do not provide FDA with a scientific justification for subjecting all bioengineered foods to such testing."[49]

The CFS is currently considering their next litigation efforts.

Citizens' Petition Against the FDA

In February 2007, three advocacy organizations—the Cancer Prevention Coalition, the Organic Consumers Association, and Family Farm Defenders—filed a citizens' petition to the FDA for the withdrawal of approval for Monsanto's Posilac, a trademarked synthetic rBGH product, registered with the U.S. Patent and Trademark Office and approved by the FDA.

Recombinant bovine growth hormone, or rBGH, is also referred to as "rBST" or "BST," a bioengineered growth hormone called recombinant bovine somatotropin. The GE synthetic hormone was developed and is marketed by Monsanto under the brand name Posilac; its purpose is to boost milk production in cows artificially.

The GE hormone continues to be used at a time when the United States already reels from a surplus of milk. Retail prices of dairy products do not go down in response to an increased oversupply because, in reality, the federal government is committed to buy surplus milk. U.S. taxpayers dole out more than $300 million annually to subsidize dairy prices.[50]

As noted in his 1998 book *MILK: The Deadly Poison* and on his www.notmilk.com Web site, Robert Cohen has investigated how billions of industry dollars have been spent to influence the FDA and Congress, as well as the scientific and medical establishment. Cohen reported that when he learned in 1994 that laboratory animals got cancer from rBGH, he discovered that Monsanto fraudulently reported data, miscited references, lied about test results, and even bribed Congress. Cohen also said the FDA admitted to not reviewing important test data that showed adverse health effects; however, to protect the fledgling biotech industry, the agency approved the drug, characterizing rBGH milk as "indistinguishable" from untreated milk, even when studies have shown differences.

To convince critics that the GE drug was safe and that it would be destroyed through pasteurization, Monsanto conducted a study in Canada. A Canadian scientist, who worked with two Monsanto scientists, pasteurized milk at the normal temperature and time to prove that pasteurization would destroy rBGH. When it did not, he then pasteurized milk for thirty minutes (typically, a product is only pasteurized at a high temperature for fifteen seconds). However, thirty minutes later, only 19% of the rBGH was destroyed. When that did not work, he released powdered rBGH into milk and then pasteurized that. Finally, 90% of the "spiked milk" was destroyed, and the FDA then concluded that rBGH milk was safe to drink because "pasteurization destroyed the synthetic hormone."[51]

The petition against the FDA requests the immediate suspension of approval of Posilac based on imminent hazard and cites a section of the Federal Food, Drug, and Cosmetic Act requesting the commissioner of the FDA to label milk and other dairy products produced with the use of Posilac with a cancer risk warning.[52]

In the United States, rBGH is injected into cows to increase the production of milk, but it can also create higher-than-normal levels of insulin-like growth factor-1 (IGF-1) in humans. IGF-1 is a cancer promoter that occurs naturally in the human bloodstream at normal levels; however, published research in leading scientific journals has linked elevated levels of IGF-1 to increased risk of breast and prostate cancers.

The petition is also based on other abnormalities in the composition of rBGH milk resulting from toxicity in animals. Also deemed "cow crack," the biweekly rBGH shots force cows to produce approximately 15-20% more milk for a few years but milk production declines after that. In the meantime, cow udders swell, and they develop painful, bloody sores from an infection called mastitis. To counter the high levels of mastitis, cows are then given large doses of antibiotics. As a side effect of Posilac, cows have been known to suffer from shortened life spans, increased birth defects, and high rates of diseases, infertility, and stress.[53] Not surprisingly, Monsanto also manufactures antibiotics and tranquilizers to sell to farmers whose cows have been injected with their rBGH.

Considerable light has been shone on rBGH by Samuel S. Epstein, M.D., chair of the Cancer Prevention Coalition, professor emeritus of environmental and occupational medicine at the School of Public Health at the University of Illinois at Chicago. Epstein is an internationally recognized authority on the causes and prevention of cancer, including carcinogenic ingredients and contaminants in food and other consumer products. He is the author of, among others, the new book *What's in Your Milk? An Exposé of Industry and Government Cover-Up on the Dangers of the Genetically Engineered (rBGH) Milk You're Drinking*. To read the nine-page citizens' petition in its entirety, go to www.preventcancer.com/publications/pdf/Petition_Posilac_feb157.pdf.

The impact of rBGH on public health is astounding when you realize that in 2004 the average American consumed 591 pounds of dairy products.[54]

As more factual scientific information becomes available and public understanding grows, public interest groups such as the Organic Consumers Association and the Oregon Physicians for Social Responsibility have helped increase awareness of the health risks of rBGH. As a result, consumers have increasingly demanded rBGH-free milk.

In 2005, the Tillamook County Creamery Association's dairy farmers banned the use of Monsanto's Posilac. Tillamook is Oregon's most productive dairy cooperative and one of the state's best-known brands. Tillamook, founded in 1909, had $262 million in sales in 2003. They based their decision on increasing inquiries by consumers over the use of the hormone. In November 2004, a Monsanto representative wrote a letter to the company, asserting that Tillamook's decision was ill-advised and would reduce member dairies' profits.[55]

"I think this is a confirmation that our members believe in us," said Christie Lincoln, association spokesperson for Tillamook. "We are a consumer-driven company, so we're keeping consumers in mind." Lincoln also said the dairy association had been under pressure from Monsanto to withdraw the proposed ban by sending its attorneys to Oregon to propose an amendment to association bylaws to prevent the ban. Rick North, spokesperson for Oregon Physicians for Social Responsibility, called the Tillamook ban a victory for consumers. "They're not only doing the right thing, they're doing the smart thing," North said of the co-op vote. "This should be great for their business."[56]

Among others, Ben & Jerry's Homemade, Inc., Stonyfield Farm, Alta Dena, Organic Valley Family of Farms, and Brown Cow Farm have pledged to go rBGH-free. Similarly, Starbucks announced it would shift to rBGH-free milk products. Safeway also said it would reduce use of some milk brands that use rBGH, and Dean Foods, the nation's largest milk processor and distributor, has also begun demanding rBGH-free milk.

How has Monsanto responded to decreasing sales of Posilac? In 2007, the corporation announced a study to "prove" that consumers are being misled by claims that milk from cows not treated with Posilac is safer or more healthful than rBGH milk. They had 213 samples from ninety-five milk brands collected from forty-eight states analyzed, using third-party testing facilities and an independent auditing firm. According to Monsanto, the analysis found no difference in concentrations of antibiotic residues, IGF-1, progesterone, or nutrients in the milk samples tested.

Here's the rub: not all conventionally produced milk contains rBGH. Monsanto did not determine if any of the milk used in their comparisons actually came from cows that received Posilac. Monsanto did nothing to determine the origin of the milk they tested, so they have no way to know how much, if any, of that milk came from cows injected with Posilac. "To pull milk off the shelves without even knowing the origin of the milk or knowing whether the cows were treated with Posilac or not and call it a scientific study is laughable," said Center for Food Safety spokesperson Charles Margulis.[57]

The government spends millions of taxpayer dollars to buy unused milk and dairy products, one of the biggest forms of subsidies; meanwhile, the FDA and Monsanto contaminate the U.S. dairy supply with a GE hormone banned almost everywhere else in the world.

CONTINUING TO GAMBLE WITH YOUR HEALTH

The biotechnology industry, food manufacturers, and U.S. government agencies continue to claim that GE foods are safe, even though none of them have been safety tested for human consumption. "Nobody's been able to prove that anyone has ever gotten sick from GE foods" is a common chant of biotech proponents.

Most Americans have not worried about GE food because they trust the regulatory system; however, in the United States there is no system to track health problems caused by GE food. Corporations developing GE food may volunteer to send data to the FDA but there is no official approval required before it ends up in American grocery stores. "It's left up to the good nature of Monsanto or DuPont or other companies to do the right thing," said Gregory Jaffe, director of the biotechnology project at Center for Science in the Public Interest. [58]

Trusting companies that have repeatedly done business at the expense of public health to reprogram the world's food supply is risky. No one knows what will happen as a result of long-term consumption of GE food; however, in addition to cancer concerns, scientists have expressed concerns about horizontal gene transfer, allergies, and other potential illnesses.

Horizontal Gene Transfer

Dr. Mae-Wan Ho is the director of the UK-based Institute of Science in Society, scientific advisor to Third World Network, scientific advisor and editor of *Science in Society* magazine, and is on the Independent Science Panel, which consists of prominent scientists committed to the promotion of science for the public good. She formerly headed the Bio-Electrodynamics laboratory at the UK Open University with more than thirty-five years of experience in research and teaching. One of her concerns about genetic engineering has been horizontal gene transfer, which is any process in which an organism transfers genetic material to another species by processes similar to infection. For example, human genes have been transferred into pigs, sheep, fish, rice, and bacteria, and fish genes have been transferred into potatoes. As a result, completely new, unnatural genes are in our food supply.

When scientists isolate a gene from one type of organism and shoot it into the DNA of another species, they disrupt its natural functioning. Because the transplanted gene is foreign to its new surroundings, it cannot adequately function without an artificial boost, or promoter. That is done by taking the section of DNA and fusing it to a pathogenic virus before insertion. Dr. Ho says the virus changes the behavior of the transplanted gene and causes it to function like an invading virus, very different from the way it behaves within its native organism and from the way the engineered organism's own genes behave.[59]

One viral promoter that is used in most GE plants comes from the cauliflower mosaic virus (CaMV), which is closely related to the human hepatitis-B virus. Because all genes contain dormant viruses, there is a potential for the CaMV promoter to reactivate them, and it may also have effects on host genes far away from the site of foreign gene insertion.[60] To manipulate, replicate, and transfer genes, scientists use recombined versions of those same genetic parasites that cause diseases in humans, such as cancers and others that carry and spread virulence genes and antibiotic-resistance genes. Therefore, according to Dr. Ho, the technology "will contribute to an increase in the frequency of horizontal gene transfer of those genes that are responsible for virulence and antibiotic resistance and allow them to recombine to generate new pathogens."[61]

Allergies

After GE soy was introduced into England, soy allergies increased by 50%; however, because GE foods are labeled in the European Union, allergies have been tracked. "All fifteen countries in the EU require labeling. The reason U.S. companies have fought against labeling; it's not just about choice, it's because if there's no tracking, they can't get a database of health effects," said Andrew Kimbrell, Center for Food Safety.[62]

A well-known case that demonstrates the validity of this concern surfaced when the once-available nutritional supplement tryptophan was banned by the FDA in 1990 due to an outbreak of Eosinophilia-Myalgia Syndrome (EMS). EMS is a blood disease that is usually associated with parasitic infections or severe allergies. From July 1989 to December 1990, more than 1,500 cases of EMS and thirty-eight deaths were associated with the outbreak in the United States.[63]

However, in a report released by the Centers for Disease Control (CDC) in August 1992, researchers revealed that tryptophan was *not* the cause of the EMS outbreak. The CDC, working with scientists from the Mayo Clinic, the Oregon State Health Division, and the Minnesota Department of Health traced the cause of the EMS crisis to tryptophan manufactured by a single Japanese company, Showa Denka.[64] The Japanese company had genetically engineered bacteria that could produce higher amounts of tryptophan than the non-GE version.

Because the batch of tryptophan that had been made from GE bacteria had not been labeled any differently than non-GE tryptophan, it was not apparent that Showa Denka's GE tryptophan was the cause of the outbreak.[65] The FDA has never publicly admitted that the GE tryptophan was the cause of the EMS outbreak, yet all tryptophan remains banned in the United States today.

It is critical to note that the assessment of the allergenicity of a GE food crop is difficult to determine when the gene is transferred from a source not eaten before. In the absence of reliable methods for allergy testing, it is, according to Dr. Arpad Pusztai, "impossible to definitely establish whether a new GM crop is allergenic or not before its release into the human/animal food/feed chain."[66]

Illnesses

CDC figures that were reported at the end of 1999 showed a two- to ten-fold rise in food-related illnesses compared with 1994, when GE food was introduced into the food supply. The CDC stated, "Food is responsible for twice the number of illnesses in the U.S. [in 2001] as scientists thought just seven years ago ... At least 80% of food-related illnesses are caused by viruses or other pathogens that scientists cannot even identify."[67]

CDC estimates from 2005 revealed that 76 million Americans get sick, more than 300,000 are hospitalized, and 5,000 people die from foodborne illnesses each year. Known pathogens account for only approximately 14 million illnesses, 60,000 hospitalizations, and 1,800 deaths annually.[68] Yet biotech proponents continue to insist that there is no evidence that GE food has ever caused any harm.[69] Laws in America make it impossible to track the source of such illnesses or have a reliable database for health concerns.

When the biotech industry claims there is no evidence of adverse health effects from GE foods, one might ask to which scientific studies they are referring. What is known, at the very least, is that the consumption of GE food has coincided in the United States with an increase in reported food-related illnesses and allergies.[70]

SCIENTISTS' OPEN LETTER
ON THE HAZARDS OF GENETICALLY
ENGINEERED FOODS AND CROPS

Released by Dr. Dominique Beroule on behalf of the Joint International GM Opposition Day coordinating committee, the following letter was read during the international video conference and used at related demonstrations (April 2006 in Chicago and in Brussels).

The current generation of genetically modified (GM) crops unnecessarily risks the health of the population and the environment. Present knowledge is not sufficient to safely and predictably modify the plant genome, and the risks of serious side effects far outweigh the benefits. We urge you to stop feeding the products of

---

this infant science to our population and ban the release of these crops into the environment where they can never be recalled.

The current technology was rushed to market long before the science was worked out. Its introduction was accompanied with rigged research, bribes, gagged scientists, cover-ups, and regulatory agencies stacked with industry representatives. With mounting evidence of serious health and environmental problems, we must act quickly to end the charade and this dangerous abuse of public trust.

Current safety assessments are inadequate to catch most of the harmful effects. When a foreign gene is artificially inserted into a living organism such as a GM crop, the preexisting natural gene of the organism can unintentionally be deleted, switched off, permanently switched on, mutated or fragmented. Hundreds of natural genes may change the way they generate their proteins (basic molecules that form living cells), and even the newly introduced protein may differ from what was intended.

Key assumptions used as the basis for safety claims have been overturned and several adverse findings suggest that GM foods are unsafe. GM-fed animals had problems with their growth, organ development and immune responsiveness, blood and liver cell formation, as well as damaged organs (bleeding stomachs, excessive cell growth, and inflammation in lung tissue), sterility problems, and increased death rates, including among the offspring.

Risks are increased by the fact that the genes inserted into GM food not only survive digestion, but transfer into body organs and circulation. Transgenes have been found in the blood, liver, spleen and kidneys. DNA can even travel via the placenta into the unborn. The only human clinical trial showed that transgenes from soy transfer into intestinal bacteria.

Claims that no one has gotten hurt from GM foods are misleading, since no one monitors human health impacts. We do know that soy allergies skyrocketed by 50 percent after GM soybeans were imported to the UK, and a GM food supplement killed about 100 Americans and caused 5,000-10,000 to fall sick.

Some GM crops create their own pesticide called Bt. Their approval relied on the assumption that Bt toxin is not bioactive in mammals. But Bt toxin caused powerful immune responses and abnormal and excessive cell growth in mice. Filipinos living next to Bt cornfields developed mysterious symptoms during the time of pollination—three seasons in a row—and blood tests showed an immune response to Bt. A November 2005 report from India claims that Bt cotton also creates allergic responses. What if Bt genes transfer to gut bacteria like soya genes do? They could turn our internal flora into living pesticide factories.

Despite the public relations spin, GM crops increase the use of herbicides, lower average yield, and endanger food security. They are detrimental to sustainable and organic farming, and trap farmers in a cycle of indebtedness and dependence. They endanger biodiversity, harm beneficial insects, damage soil bacteria, contaminate non-GM varieties and may persist in the environment for generations. Insurance companies do not want to cover the risks inherent in GMOs. Consumers do not want them.

Please act today to protect our health, our environment, and future generations.

This letter was mainly written by Dr. Arpad Pusztai; author received permission from Dr. Arpad Pusztai and Jeffrey M. Smith to print this letter in its entirety. Source: Organic Consumers Association (December 20, 2005). www.organicconsumers.org/ ge/openletter122105.cfm.

Chapter 3
Connect These Dots

The problem with biotechnology as it's presented today is that those pushing its benefits stand to gain enormously from it ... we've learned from experience with the tobacco, nuclear, petrochemical, automobile, and pharmaceutical industries and military establishments that vested interest alone shapes a spokesperson's perspective and precludes an ability to examine criticisms or concerns in an open fashion.[1]
Dr. David Suzuki in "Biotechnology: A Geneticist's Perspective"

Monsanto was required to submit a safety report on Posilac to the FDA. Margaret Miller, one of Monsanto's researchers, put the report on rBGH together. However, shortly before her submission to the FDA, she left Monsanto and was hired by the FDA as deputy director of the Office of New Animal Drugs. One of Miller's first jobs was to determine if she should approve the report she wrote for Monsanto. She approved it.[2]
Center for Media and Democracy's "Labeling Issues, Revolving Doors, rBGH, Bribery, and Monsanto"

In 2003, George W. Bush signed a five-year, $15 billion global AIDS-relief bill for the citizens of fourteen African and Caribbean countries ... to receive assistance, the beneficiary countries must accept GE foods from the United States.[3]
John Tarleton's CorpWatch article "USA: Bush Delivers Emergency AIDS Relief to Republican Allies"

Why has the American public been excluded from the discussions and policy-making decisions on GE food? One reason could be because corporations have invested billions of dollars in biotechnology and have successfully lobbied U.S. government agencies to allow GE food to enter the American food chain and the environment without public awareness.

Support of the biotech industry is not an issue of party politics. It is simply and purely an issue of money and power. In the midst of this, what happened to the government's responsibility to protect the American public's health?

PRESIDENTIAL ADVOCACY

The lack of regulation of the biotech industry began with policies set by the Reagan Administration in the early 1980s. To establish biotech world dominance, the administration's policy ensured that regulations would not be a burden on the industry. Industrial profit, not public safety, was the administration's priority. Government officials in the Office of Management and Budget, the Departments of State and Commerce, and the White House Office of Science and Technology Policy wanted to be sure that the administration did not do anything to hinder the development of the then-fledgling biotech industry.

The George H. W. Bush Administration's President's Council on Competitiveness, chaired by Vice President Dan Quayle, joined the biotechnology industry in opposing strong regulations and close oversight by federal agencies. Quayle said that government "will ensure that biotech products will receive the same oversight as other products, instead of being hampered by unnecessary regulation."[4] The rationale for this policy was the concept of "substantial equivalence," declaring that GE food is no different than conventional food. The science journal *Nature* said substantial equivalence is a "pseudo-scientific concept ... created primarily to provide an excuse for not requiring biochemical and toxicological tests."[5]

Subsequently, the Clinton Administration continued this policy. In 1995, Monsanto's CEO Robert B. Shapiro was appointed to be on Clinton's advisory committee for Trade Policy and Negotiations. Shapiro was one of the biggest contributors of "soft money" (legal funds that are not included in the ban on corporate donations) to Bill Clinton's 1996 re-election campaign. As he began his second term, Clinton publicly lauded Monsanto in his State of the Union address in February 1997. Some of the top Clinton aides, including U.S. Trade Representative Charlene Barshevsky, Secretary of State Madeleine Albright, Secretary of Agriculture Dan Glickman, and Secretary of Commerce William Daley, all lobbied their European counterparts on Monsanto's behalf.[6]

President George W. Bush has also supported the biotech industry. In 2003, he attended and spoke at the Biotechnology Industry Organization's (BIO) eleventh annual conference, praised the industry and stated, "My administration is committed to working with your industry so that the great powers of biotechnology can serve the true interests of our nation and mankind."[7]

As the largest biotech lobby group, BIO represents more than 1,100 biotech companies (including Monsanto, Syngenta, DuPont, and Bayer), academic institutions, state biotechnology centers, and related organizations.

REVOLVING DOOR

Employees commonly move through what has been coined the "revolving door" between corporations and the public agencies that regulate them. For those concerned about the health and environmental hazards of genetic engineering, the revolving door between the biotechnology industry and federal regulating agencies is a paramount issue.

According to a study of federal records by the Center for Public Integrity, between 1998 and 2004, more than 2,200 former federal government employees registered as federal lobbyists. Records show that more than 12% of current lobbyists are former executive and legislative branch employees; more than two hundred were former members of Congress, and forty-two were former heads of governmental agencies.

James Thurber, professor of government and director of the Center for Congressional and Presidential Studies and the Campaign Management and Lobbying Institutes at American University in Washington, D.C., commented that the revolving door allows for "undue influence" by former government employees and those that can afford their services. He referred to lobbying as "a second-career option" for those leaving government, one that can be much more lucrative than working in the public sector.[8]

It is worth noting that in 2007, Congress approved themselves a pay increase of $4,400, raising their salaries to approximately $170,000 per year. This puts Congress in an income bracket above 97% of American households. This raise also comes at a time when the majority of Americans are falling behind economically.[9] It helps explain why Congress is out of touch with the American people they are supposed to represent, and why industry continues to influence public policy in its favor.

To put it into perspective, Pennsylvania Representative James Greenwood is just one example of how lucrative the private sector can be for a government official. Greenwood chaired the Congressional subcommittee that regulates the biotech and drug industries, yet he took over as BIO's president in January 2005. Greenwood accepted the BIO job in July 2004, but stayed in public office until January 2005 to finish out his government term. BIO paid Greenwood $650,000 plus $200,000 in bonuses for his help in "encouraging a regulatory climate in Washington that will help our industry."[10]

The list of individuals who have gone through the "revolving door" is both shocking and extensive. Monsanto is one company to have largely infiltrated and influenced Washington through the revolving door. Through economic and political pressure, the company has influenced past administrations' federal bureaucrats and continues to maintain prominent connections to the George W. Bush Administration. A comprehensive list can be found on The Edmonds Institute Web site at www.edmonds-institute.org.

Michael Taylor, FDA Attorney

After graduating from law school in 1976, Michael Taylor went to work for the FDA during the Carter Administration, and at one point, was staff lawyer and executive assistant to the commissioner of the FDA.

In 1981, Taylor left the FDA to be a partner in the law firm of King & Spaulding and became the firm's food and drug law (FDA) specialist, where he supervised a nine-lawyer group whose clients included Monsanto. During his ten years at King & Spaulding, Taylor represented Monsanto's efforts to gain FDA approval for Posilac (rBGH). Taylor wrote articles opposing the Delaney Clause, a 1958 federal law prohibiting the introduction of known carcinogens into processed foods, which had been opposed by Monsanto and other chemical and pesticide companies.[11]

In 1991, he left the law firm to rejoin the FDA under President George Bush, Sr., this time as deputy commissioner for policy when the agency was reviewing rBGH. It was in 1994 during the Clinton Administration that Monsanto's GE hormone, one of the most controversial drug applications in the history of the FDA, was approved under Taylor's influence.[12]

Taylor was also instrumental in writing the FDA's rBGH labeling guidelines that would prohibit dairy corporations from making any distinction between products produced with or without rBGH.[13] Just days after Taylor's policy was implemented, King & Spaulding—still representing Monsanto—filed a suit against two dairy farms that had labeled their milk rBGH-free.

In response, the Foundation for Economic Trends petitioned the FDA and the Department of Health and Human Services to investigate Taylor's conflict of interest. Three members of Congress then asked the General Accounting Office to investigate. Within days of the complaint, Taylor left the FDA to work for the USDA as the administrator of the Food Safety and Inspection Service, a position he held from 1994 to 1996.

After representing Monsanto at King & Spaulding and having worked at the FDA and the USDA, Taylor went directly to Monsanto to work as vice president of public policy in the late 1990s.

Margaret Miller, FDA Researcher

Another example of the government-industry revolving door is Margaret Miller. According to SourceWatch, a project of the Center for Media and Democracy, Margaret Miller, one of Monsanto's researchers, put together the report on rBGH. However, shortly before her submission to the FDA, she left Monsanto and was hired by the FDA as deputy director of the Office of New Animal Drugs. One of Miller's first jobs was to determine if she should approve the report she wrote for Monsanto. She approved it.[14]

Because cows injected with rBGH require more antibiotics (due to increased udder infections and other health problems), Miller, when at the FDA, adjusted the standard allowable limit of antibiotic residue from one part per *hundred million* to one part per *one million*, an arbitrary increase of one hundred times the allowable legal limit.

Suzanne Sechen, FDA Data Reviewer

Working with Miller was another Monsanto researcher, Susan Sechen, a data reviewer at the FDA between 1988 and 1990.

While conducting research for Monsanto at Cornell University in Ithaca, New York, Sechen had three temporary jobs at the FDA, developing the criteria under which rBGH would be reviewed. She did research for Monsanto on Monsanto's products and sent her results to Monsanto. One of her professors at Cornell was one of Monsanto's university consultants and was known to promote rBGH.[15]

Largely due to Monsanto's influence (Taylor, Miller, and Sechen), the FDA has never required long-term studies for rBGH. In 1994, the General Accounting Office found Margaret Miller and Susan Sechen violated ethics rules eleven times, but nothing was done about it. They were both involved with the FDA's technical review of Monsanto's rBGH and had been researchers employed by Monsanto. Even while employed at the FDA, Miller and Sechen published articles for Monsanto. As the primary data reviewer for Monsanto's rBGH application, Sechen was also in a position to review and approve her own rBGH research work.[16]

Carol Tucker Foreman, Consumer Advocate

Between 1973 and 1977, Carol Tucker Foreman was the executive director of the Consumer Federation of America's (CFA) Food Policy Institute. In April 2000, the CFA's National Food Policy Conference sponsors were the American Feed Association and the Olsson, Frank, and Weeda law firm, both proponents of the passage of "food disparagement" laws, which the American Farm Bureau Federation has lobbied into law in thirteen states. Those laws eliminate free-speech rights and impose censorship on the media regarding concerns of food safety issues.[17]

During the Carter Administration, Foreman served as assistant secretary of agriculture in charge of meat and poultry inspection at the USDA. When she left the USDA, she was president for eighteen years of a public relations and lobbying company, whose clients included Monsanto, the Beef Council, and Philip Morris. She lobbied in support of Monsanto's campaign to win approval for Posilac, and with her help, Monsanto was assured that rBGH dairy products would remain unlabeled.[18]

In May 2000, the Clinton White House appointed Foreman as the consumer advocate on the international Biotech Consultative Forum Delegation to reconcile the differences between the United States and the rest of the world on the issue of GE food. Critics of GE food, including Greenpeace, the Center for Food Safety, Friends of the Earth, the Organic Consumers Association, and Public Citizen, wanted her appointment revoked due to her close ties to Monsanto and the biotech industry.[19]

Foreman used her influence to get Virginia Weldon, Monsanto's former public relations chief, appointed to Clinton's Committee of Scientific Advisors and Gore's Sustainable Development Roundtable, groups that recommended the Delaney Clause (which said that a known carcinogen cannot be added to food) should be replaced with more "flexible" legislation.[20] Since December 2002, Foreman has been on DuPont's Biotechnology Advisory Panel.

Robert Fraley, USDA Technical Advisor

Robert Fraley was a technical advisor to the USDA, U.S. Office of Technology Assessment, U.S. Agency for International Development, the National Science Foundation, and National Academy of Science. He has been involved in agricultural biotechnology since the early 1980s and has been with Monsanto for more than twenty years, even while serving as technical advisor to the government. Currently he is executive vice president and chief technology officer for Monsanto and a member of BIO.[21]

Michael Kantor, Secretary of Commerce

Attorney Michael Kantor, who played a key role in President Bill Clinton's 1992 election campaign, was the U.S. trade representative during Clinton's first term and then secretary of commerce from 1996 to 1997. In May 1997, Kantor left his government position to work with his previous law firm Mayer, Brown, & Platt (Mayer, Brown, Rowe, & Maw as of 2003) and to be on Monsanto's board of directors. The law firm has been on the side of protecting Monsanto's interests in matters of international trade, food safety, and product labeling. Kantor pushed the Clinton administration to pressure the European Union to purchase Monsanto's GE grain.[22]

L. Val Giddings, USDA Regulatory Division

For five years, Giddings contributed to and directed biotechnology policy studies for the Office of Technology Assessment and was then a biotechnology consultant to the World Bank. From 1989 to 1997, he was senior staff geneticist, international team leader, and branch chief for science and policy coordination with the biotechnology products regulatory division of the USDA. While at the USDA, Giddings represented the U.S. government at the first meeting of the Ad Hoc Working Group on Biosafety Protocol. Giddings left the USDA and became vice president for food and agriculture of the Biotechnology Industry Organization.[23] He attended the second meeting as the representative of the biotech industry.

Rodney Sippel, Federal Judge

Rodney Sippel worked for the law firm now known as Husch & Eppenberger from 1981 to 1993, when he left to serve as an administrative aide to Missouri Representative Richard A. Gephardt. He rejoined the law firm in 1995 and was listed as an attorney on a 1997-98 case representing Monsanto in a civil lawsuit against seed company Pioneer Hi-Bred International. While still listed as a Monsanto attorney, Sippel was nominated by President Bill Clinton in 1997 to fill a vacancy at the federal courthouse in St. Louis, Missouri (Monsanto's home city and state). His name was not removed as a Monsanto attorney until 1998, even though he concurrently was a federal judge.[24]

In 2003 and 2004, Sippel presided over a price-fixing case, where he ruled in favor of Monsanto and other seed companies by denying the lawsuit class-action status. In another case in 2003, Sippel awarded Monsanto $2.9 million in damages from a Tennessee farmer accused of violating Monsanto's patent.[25]

Marcia Hale, Governmental Affairs Director

Marcia Hale was political director of the Democratic Congressional Campaign Committee, former assistant to President Clinton, and director for intergovernmental affairs, which is a liaison between the White House and state and local governments. She left her government position to be Monsanto's director of international governmental affairs, in charge of coordinating Monsanto's public affairs and corporate strategy in the UK and Ireland.[26] Hale is now with the Washington, D.C. law firm McKenna Long & Aldridge, focusing on local, state, and governmental affairs.

Ann Veneman, USDA Secretary of Agriculture

During the George H. W. Bush Administration, Veneman served as associate administrator of the foreign agricultural service, deputy undersecretary for international affairs and commodity programs, and as deputy secretary at the USDA. Later, she was the USDA's secretary of agriculture during the George W. Bush Administration from 2001 to 2005.

Between her job at the USDA under President George H. W. Bush and becoming the USDA's secretary of agriculture under President George W. Bush in 2001, Veneman was director of the biotech company Calgene, which was the first company to bring GE food—the Flavr Savr tomato—to supermarket shelves (Calgene is now owned by Monsanto). She served on the International Food and Agricultural Trade Policy Council, a group funded by Monsanto, Syngenta, Cargill, Nestle, Kraft, Grocery Manufacturers of America, and others.[27]

In 2005, Veneman, who was nominated by President George W. Bush, became executive director of the United Nations Children's Fund (UNICEF), the U.N. agency responsible for protecting children's health, welfare, and rights.

John Nichols wrote about her nomination in *The Nation* and quoted Ravi Narayan, coordinator for the global secretariat of the People's Health Movement, in a 2005 letter to U.N. Secretary-General Kofi Annan and the members of the executive board of UNICEF: "Ms. Veneman's training and experience as a corporate lawyer for agribusiness do not qualify her for the substantial task of leading the agency most responsible for the rights of children worldwide ... Indeed, her performance ... has been characterized by the elevation of corporate profit above people's right to food."[28]

John Ashcroft, Attorney General

Ashcroft was chosen as President George W. Bush's Attorney General (AG) from 2001 to 2005. Prior to his position as AG, Ashcroft was a senator who led calls to the Clinton Administration to promote GE crops in developing countries and to persuade Europe to accept them. Ashcroft was the top recipient of Monsanto contributions when he tried to get re-elected to the U.S. Senate. Even though he did not get re-elected, he was appointed President George W. Bush's Attorney General instead.[29] Today, Ashcroft is building a consulting business working with security and other firms to find business with federal agencies.

Tommy Thompson, Secretary of Health and Human Services

Tommy Thompson, secretary of Health and Human Services from 2001 to 2005, oversaw food safety, pharmaceuticals, and the FDA.

Prior to serving as secretary of Health and Human Services, he received $50,000 in donations from Monsanto during his winning campaign for Wisconsin governor. He used state funds to set up a $37 million biotech zone in Wisconsin and was one of thirteen state governors to launch a campaign, partly funded by Monsanto, to persuade Americans of the benefits of GE crops.[30]

Clarence Thomas, Supreme Court Judge

Clarence Thomas was Monsanto's lawyer before he was appointed Supreme Court judge in 1991 by President George H. W. Bush.[31]

Linda J. Fisher, EPA Deputy Administrator

Attorney Linda Fisher has been involved in environmental issues throughout her career. In her experience at the EPA from 1983 to 1993, she held many high-level positions, including chief of staff, assistant administrator for policy, planning and evaluation, and assistant administrator for prevention, pesticides, and toxic substances.

From 1995 to 2000, she was vice president of governmental affairs for Monsanto, heading their Washington, D.C., lobbying office until she was nominated by President George W. Bush in 2001 to be the EPA's second-in-command as deputy administrator. In 2004, Fisher joined DuPont and is currently vice president and chief sustainability officer.[32]

LOBBYISTS

Worldwide, approximately two hundred corporations—eighty-two of them based in the United States and most with revenues larger than many national economies—control over a quarter of the world's economy.[33] Corporations increase their power in the marketplace by financially supporting political candidates and public officials. Many of the people who go through the revolving door become lobbyists who play a significant role in influencing public policy.

Monsanto paid out more than $22.5 million in lobbying dollars from 1998 through 2004. Their lobbyists work to affect regulations that apply to its GE crops, to open European and other foreign markets for GE food, and to win legislation that can shape the federal agriculture budget to benefit the corporation. In 2005, Monsanto had nine in-house Washington lobbyists on its payroll and another thirteen at private firms.[34]

State lobbyists and the companies that hire them spent more than $1 billion in 2005 to influence state lawmakers and officials. Working across the nation were approximately forty thousand registered lobbyists paid to advance the agendas of almost fifty thousand companies and organizations, which averaged more than five lobbyists per state legislator. Lobby spending was nearly $953 million in 2004 and increased by 22% in 2005, totaling $1.16 billion.[35]

While many other governmental disclosure forms are filed with agencies like the Federal Election Commission and the Office of Government Ethics, lobby disclosure forms are filed with the House and the Senate. This creates conflicts of interest because members of Congress often leave public office to work for private lobbying firms. It also puts Congress in charge of monitoring their former colleagues and employees, which could negatively affect the possibility of a potential lobby career for any whistleblowers.[36]

The Center for Public Integrity's figures from 1998 to 2004 show that the Biotechnology Industry Organization (BIO) spent $23.6 million in lobbying dollars, with $5.1 million of that amount spent in 2004 alone. Established in July 1993 and based in Washington, D.C., BIO has grown from sixteen employees and a $2.1 million budget to almost a one hundred-member staff with a $40 million budget by 2004. The organization's Web site states that the goal of a biotechnology company is to "build a revenue and profit-generating business." The Center for Responsive Politics says the organization's lobbying priorities are promoting GE food, blocking government price controls of biotech drugs, streamlining the regulatory process for biotech products, and supporting tax incentives for the industry.[37]

As the biotech industry's major trade association, BIO represents large and small companies as well as academic and research centers that use biotechnology to develop medical, agricultural, industrial, and environmental products. BIO's members are not only in the United States but also in thirty-three other countries. Board of directors members include Hugh Grant, current president and CEO of Monsanto, J. Erik Fyrwald, group vice president of DuPont Biotechnology, Susan Desmond-Hellmann, president of product development of biotech company Genentech, and W. Pete Siggelko, vice president of plant genetics and biotechnology of Dow AgroSciences.[38]

BIO has been quick to dismiss research that questions the risks of GE crops. When Dr. Arpad Pusztai was fired from the Rowett Institute after he had raised questions about the safety of GE food, L. Val Giddings, on behalf of BIO, applauded Pusztai's dismissal and said to *Biotechnology Newswatch*, an industry journal, "This is a study that should never have seen the light of day."[39]

TAXPAYERS BANKROLL BIOTECH

Being financially under the influence of the biotech industry, with all of the inherent conflicts of interest, the U.S. government—funded by taxpayers—heavily invests in and promotes the biotech industry in the United States and abroad.

U.S. Government Owns Biotech Patents

According to the USDA's Economic Research Service database from 1976 to 2000, the U.S. government owns 421 patents, which include plant technologies, metabolic pathways and biological processes in plants and animals, biological control of plants and animals, and more.

The USDA has spent hundreds of thousands of taxpayer dollars to develop "terminator technology," which, when used, makes it impossible for farmers to save seeds for replanting. Although part of the USDA's mission is to support American farmers, this technology is in direct opposition to a farmer's right to save seeds from one year to the next. A major concern about "terminator technology" is that traits from GE crops can contaminate non-GE crops, making most or all of the seeds in a region sterile. Despite public concerns, the USDA continues to pursue the sterilization technology with its industry partners and as of 2000, the U.S. government owned seven patents on "terminator technology."[40]

R&D Funding

One of the largest taxpayer subsidies to the biotech industry is via research and development funds. The U.S. government has allocated more than $120 *billion* annually to support R&D in laboratories, colleges and universities, private firms, and other locations. This money is distributed among twenty-two agencies of the federal government; however, only six federal agencies control 95% of these funds: the Department of Defense, the Department of Health and Human Services (of which the FDA is a part), the National Aeronautics and Space Administration, the Department of Energy, the National Science Foundation, and the USDA.[41]

Federal-government support for biotech has three major components: the funding of basic research mostly conducted at university laboratories and research institutes; the funding of R&D activities at federal and state agencies, which use part of these funds for research outside their laboratories; and programs created to increase the productivity of U.S. firms by facilitating the use of new technologies.[42]

The National Institutes of Health (NIH) has typically funded biological research in the United States. It is the primary biomedical research division of the

Department of Health and Human Services and allocates about three-fourths of its public funds for biotechnology activities.[43] Several of the industry's top scientists were trained at NIH, and many private companies have grown out of federally funded (NIH) university research.

Much of biotech research is conducted in each state at land-grant colleges, which were set up in the nineteenth century specifically to support agricultural research. According to a Web site created by a group of land-grant colleges, one of their goals is to "make information on agricultural biotechnology available to the public and to participate in the dialogue about the benefits and risks of this new technology, which fast is becoming a part of our everyday lives."[44]

According to the 2004 report *Vital Assets: Federal Investment in Research and Development at the Nation's Universities and Colleges*, approximately two-thirds of federal funds allocated to universities and colleges for R&D is focused on only one field of science—life science—and federal R&D funding is granted to select research universities. The 189-page study "raises questions about whether other national needs (such as environment, energy, homeland security, and education) are receiving the investment they require and whether the concentration of dollars at a few institutions is shortchanging science students at institutions that receive little or no federal R&D funding."[45]

Today, each state has federal- and state-funded (taxpayer-funded) programs to grow biotechnology businesses and offer a supportive public policy. Support strategies to boost biotech business, among others, include tax breaks, free workforce training, funds and financial incentives, and business startup support.[46] The survey, *State Government Initiatives in Biotechnology 2001*, found that forty-one of the forty-eight states that responded had initiatives to support the development of biotechnology. These initiatives include investments in research, education, and technology infrastructure, and various policies and programs to improve the climate for biotechnology startup businesses.[47] The benefits to corporations are immeasurable, yet they do not show up as direct subsidies to any particular company.

For example, New Jersey established three biotechnology research centers. In 1995, legislation authorized state agencies to provide financial assistance for the construction of biotechnology research facilities, allowing the use of pension funds to be invested in new firms and prohibiting local governments from regulating industry activities at all.[48]

The biotech center in North Carolina was a substantial investment by that state's government and one that has paid high dividends since the $5 million grant that created it in 1981. Since being spun off as a nonprofit corporation in 1984, it had received $139 million from the state as of 2003, which was 90% of its total revenue.[49] The Commerce Finance Center, part of the North Carolina Department of Commerce, coordinates financial incentives that apply to biotech and other industries. These include the governor's industrial recruitment fund, tax credits for job creation, and free biotech workforce training at community colleges. The North Carolina recruitment fund helps companies that are creating jobs and investing in new machinery and equipment. Grants range from $50,000 to $1 million, and $15 million went into the fund in fiscal year 2001.[50]

Indiana offers financial incentives for biotechnology. Energize Indiana is the state's ten-year, $1.25-billion plan to create 200,000 high-wage, high-skilled jobs in the life sciences and other high-tech fields. Energize Indiana's Indiana Venture Fund is a ten-year, $144-million investment that allows companies to leverage state money to help biotech startups get off the ground.[51]

To create Michigan's Life Sciences Corridor, both Dow and Pharmacia (formerly Monsanto) partnered with Michigan State University and the University of Michigan, while the state legislature allocated $50 million annually for twenty years of all of the state's revenues from tobacco settlement funds to universities, research institutions, and the biotech industry.[52]

In 2003, the Minneapolis, Minnesota legislature approved a five thousand-acre tax-free zone for biotechnology and health science firms, which pay no state corporate income, property or sales taxes, and investors pay no state capital gains taxes. Companies also receive job creation and R&D tax credits. The state allocated $2 million toward a new biotechnology center, with a five-year goal of $100 million in capital from the state for the project. It is to be operated jointly by the University of Minnesota and the Mayo Clinic.[53]

The Danforth Plant Science Center in Missouri (the home of Monsanto), dedicated to plant biotechnology research, received a $50-million donation from the Monsanto Foundation and $25 million in state tax credits. Located near

Monsanto's headquarters, the center's discoveries are patented and licensed to the private sector, while individual research projects draw funding mostly from taxpayer sources.[54] Monsanto's president and CEO is trustee of the Danforth Center.

In 1999, Monsanto considered sending its subsidiary Integrated Protein Technologies (IPT) from Missouri to either North Carolina or Virginia. IPT is involved in research with genetically engineering crops to make pharmaceuticals. To keep the company in the state, the Missouri Department of Economic Development offered space at a new research park on conservation land and allowed Monsanto to sell (transfer) to IPT about $4.5 million in tax credits that it had accumulated but was unable to use. The tax credits were to go toward funding research at the University of Missouri.[55] University scientists and administrators met with IPT officials to discuss potential research topics, which, among others, included "public acceptance," "media," and "marketing" of biotechnology.[56]

Crop Subsidies

GE crops have caused an economic disaster for farmers in the United States, according to a report released by Britain's Soil Association in 2002. *How to Lose Money on the Farm* was compiled from data showing how GE crops have cost American taxpayers billions in farm subsidies. "Within a few years of the introduction of GE crops, almost the entire $300 million annual U.S. maize [corn] exports to the EU had disappeared, and the U.S. share of the soy market had decreased," the report stated. In addition, the study revealed that GE crops have led to an increased use of pesticides, while resulting in overall lower crop yields.[57]

American taxpayers paid $164.7 billion in farm subsidies from 1995 to 2005 and $21 billion in 2006 alone; however, according to the Census of Agriculture, 66% of all farmers do not collect government subsidy payments because they do not grow one of the five crops that account for more than 90% of the subsidy payments in any given year (rice, wheat, corn, cotton, and soybeans). Among subsidy recipients, the large "agribusiness" farms collect almost all of the money. In fact, from 1995 to 2005, the top 10% of recipients were paid 73% of all USDA subsidies, amounting to $120.5 billion.[58]

It is shocking, albeit not surprising, that large agribusinesses receive billions in federal subsidy support year after year. There are no limits on the subsidies a large agribusiness can receive. At the same time, instead of imposing a limit on tax-payer subsidies to the very largest, government-dependent businesses, funds and food assistance programs for the poor get eliminated. For instance, in October 2005, the House Agriculture Committee approved a budget measure to eliminate three hundred thousand people from the Food Stamp Program,[59] while rejecting the proposed limitation of annual subsidies to $250,000 per "farm."

Continuing politics as usual (i.e. satisfying large agribusinesses), in July 2007, House Speaker Nancy Pelosi signed off on a five-year farm bill that would keep multi-billion-dollar subsidies flowing primarily to corn, soybeans, cotton, wheat, and rice. Many of these are GE crops. The bill would grant subsidies to farmers earning up to $1 million—five times more than the cap sought by the Bush Administration. According to Carolyn Lochhead's article *Pelosi Takes Heat for OK of Farm Bill*, Pelosi's motivation is to "preserve the re-election prospects of freshman Democrats in rural districts who toppled Republicans in November and helped secure Democrats their House majority and Pelosi the speakership. Nine of the freshmen sit on the House Agriculture Committee. Several said they feared any vote to reform farm programs would endanger their political prospects."[60]

Rice and Soy Subsidies

The Environmental Working Group (EWG) is a nonprofit environmental research organization and an information provider for public interest groups and concerned citizens. EWG's Farm Subsidy Database reveals that from 1995 to 2004, Riceland Foods and Producers Rice Mill in Arkansas were the top two recipients of all taxpayer-funded subsidies during those ten years, with $534 million and $295 million respectively.[61]

Riceland Foods, the top subsidy recipient, is a rice miller and marketer and soybean producer, with most of the soy GE. Previous president and CEO of Riceland Richard Bell came to Riceland after serving as the assistant agriculture secretary for international affairs and commodity programs in the U.S. government. He also served as president of the USDA's Commodity Credit Corporation (CCC), an organization that decides which subsidized crops will be bought and sent abroad as foreign food aid.[62] Under Richard Bell, Riceland sold $5 million worth of rice to Iraq in a food-for-crude exchange, the first American rice sent to Iraq since international sanctions were imposed. Riceland also shipped twenty tons of rice to Guantanamo, Cuba.[63]

If a particular commodity is overproduced by farmers, the CCC will buy a certain quantity to remove the surplus from the market. While the U.S. taxpayers heavily fund Riceland, a huge surplus of soy and rice has been grown. Aid agencies like the U.S. Agency for International Development and private volunteer organizations place orders with the CCC, which runs the requests through an approval process. The CCC allows U.S.-based farms and corporations to bid, and the contract is awarded to the lowest bidder.[64]

Considering that U.S. taxpayers have handed out more than half a billion dollars to Riceland in subsidies, it is easy to understand how they can be the lowest bidder on foreign-aid programs. Richard Bell knew this process well, having been president of the CCC as well as assistant agriculture secretary for international affairs and commodity programs before working at Riceland.

Daniel Kennedy, Richard Bell's successor, came to Riceland after serving as vice president of North American markets for Monsanto for more than sixteen years. According to a USDA publication published in 2004, Riceland expected record sales of more than $950 million in 2004. Total assets and member equity were also expected to set new records by the year's end.[65]

Riceland is not in trouble, yet American taxpayers, through the USDA, continue to pay Riceland more money in subsidies each year than to any other company. At the same time, small farms continue to go out of business because they do not qualify for subsidies.

Dairy Subsidies

Dairy subsidies in the United States totaled $3.1 billion from 1995 to 2004.[66] Why is it that Monsanto markets its Posilac as a way to radically increase milk yields with the U.S. government's (i.e., taxpayer) support? Retail prices of dairy products do not go down due to an oversupply. In fact, the federal government is committed to buy surplus milk at a high cost to taxpayers. Each year, U.S. taxpayers hand out approximately $300 million to buy surplus milk to subsidize dairy prices.

Corn Subsidies

U.S. taxpayers paid $41.9 billion in corn subsidies from 1995 to 2004. In November 2005, Iowa harvested its second-largest corn crop in history, much of it GE. One Iowa farmer had to cope with the most visible challenge arising from the growing farm subsidy program: 2.7 million bushels of corn, more than sixty-feet high and as wide as a football field. The excess corn exemplified the growth in production by American farmers in recent years, which depresses prices and raises subsidy payments.[67]

At the end of October 2005, the USDA raised its projection of corn subsidies in 2005 to $22.7 billion, up from $13.3 billion in 2004. "We are still in a condition of grossly overproducing for what the market can pay, at least what the market can pay that is acceptable to our corn producers," said Ken Cook, president of the Environmental Working Group. "We can't make up the difference in the export market [most countries will not accept U.S. GE corn], and the taxpayers are on the hook."[68]

Foreign Aid or Biotech Industry Aid?

U.S. taxpayer dollars are being used for foreign assistance programs to subsidize the export of GE products to the third world and to finance GE research.

The U.S. food industry has had trouble exporting products containing GE ingredients, so the U.S. government has turned foreign countries into alternative markets for GE products, particularly through foreign-assistance food-aid programs. More than two million tons of GE foods are sent every year to developing countries via U.S. foreign assistance.[69]

During negotiations on the Cartagena Biosafety Protocol in 2002—part of a United Nations sponsored international agreement to control and document the movement of GE crops around the world—African countries made it clear that they did not want to become a dumping ground for GE food.[70] However, because the U.S. government does not require labeling of GE products, not only is GE food produced and consumed in the United States without the American public's knowledge, but biotech foods are also being exported as food aid, at times without recipient governments' knowledge.

USAID

Funded by taxpayers, the United States Agency for International Development (USAID) is the principal U.S. agency that provides economic and humanitarian assistance to developing countries. U.S. foreign assistance has always had the advancement of America's foreign policy interests in mind, including furthering U.S. economic growth, agriculture, and trade. According to the U.S. State Department, nearly 80% of all USAID contracts and grants go directly to American firms. Foreign-assistance programs have helped create major markets for agricultural goods, new markets for American industrial exports, and have meant hundreds of thousands of jobs for Americans.[71]

President George W. Bush increased the USAID budget specifically to encourage biotechnology. Subsequently, the agency launched a $100 million program for taking biotechnology to developing countries. According to their Web site, USAID's "training and awareness raising programs" provide companies such as Monsanto, Syngenta, and Pioneer Hi-Bred with opportunities for technology transfer and "enhance public knowledge and acceptance of biotechnology."[72]

USAID has also played a leading role in promoting the acceptance of GE crops in Kenya, particularly with a GE sweet-potato project associated with the Kenyan scientist Florence Wambugu, who was recruited by Monsanto. USAID money paid for Wambugu's three-year post-doctoral position with Monsanto.[73]

Iraq Reconstruction

GRAIN is an international non-governmental organization that promotes sustainable management and use of agricultural biodiversity based on peoples' control over genetic resources and local knowledge. According to the article *Iraq's New Patent Law: A Declaration of War Against Farmers* in their February 2005 e-newsletter *Against the Grain,* when former Coalition Provisional Authority administrator L. Paul Bremer III left Baghdad after the "transfer of sovereignty" in June 2004, he left behind one hundred orders that he had enacted as chief of the occupation authority in Iraq.

Among them is Order 81, making it illegal for Iraqi farmers to re-use seeds harvested from new varieties registered under the law. The law facilitates the establishment of a new seed market in Iraq where multinational corporations can sell their seeds. While the Iraqi constitution has prohibited private ownership of biological resources, the new U.S. patent law for Iraq introduces a system of ownership of seeds, which promotes the penetration of Iraqi agriculture by large corporations.

The new law will actually facilitate the penetration of Iraqi agriculture by companies such as Monsanto, Syngenta, Bayer, and Dow Chemical. Eliminating competition from farmers is necessary for these companies to open up operations in Iraq, which the new law has achieved.[74]

AIDS Relief Bill

In June 2003, to much fanfare, President George W. Bush signed a five-year, $15 billion global AIDS-relief bill for the citizens of fourteen African and Caribbean countries. Besides giving Bush a public relations boost, the measure seemed to be of more help to U.S. pharmaceutical companies and the biotech industry than to the citizens covered by the initiative. The catch? To receive any assistance at all, the beneficiary countries had to accept GE foods from the United States.[75]

Many African nations have rejected GE foods, following the EU's lead. The AIDS bill condemned African countries that have large populations of HIV- or AIDS-infected citizens and who have rejected shipments of food aid fearing that it might be genetically engineered.

U.S. taxpayers subsidize agribusiness by buying surplus GE crops and distributing them through foreign-aid programs. This helps large corporations penetrate new markets around the world. Many of the funds originally intended to assist the poor or small farmers wind up benefiting big businesses.

Plan Colombia Benefits Monsanto

Financed by the U.S. taxpayers since 2000 and as part of a foreign aid package, one of Plan Colombia's beneficiaries is Monsanto. The corporation's chemicals have been sprayed in Colombia by aircraft to destroy coca and other plants used to make illegal drugs. It is the biggest aid commitment outside of the Middle East and Afghanistan.

Unfortunately, the program endangers the ecosystems and the health of the indigenous cultures of Colombia's Amazon Basin by destroying food crops and other natural plants, as well as killing birds, mammals, and aquatic life.* Local residents in the Colombian countryside have complained of health problems as a result of being sprayed with Monsanto's Roundup Ultra herbicide. Monsanto receives taxpayer money to provide tons of Roundup Ultra, the highly concentrated and more toxic version of Roundup. "This spraying campaign is equivalent to the Agent Orange devastation of Vietnam, a disturbance the wildlife and natural ecosystems have never recovered from," said Dr. David Olson, director of the World Wildlife Fund's conservation science program in 2000.†

Colombian leaders visited Congress in 2001 to speak out against the fumigation: "The twelve indigenous [groups] have been suffering under this plague as if it were a government decree to exterminate our culture and our very survival … Our legal crops, our only sustenance—manioc, banana, palms, sugar cane, and corn—have been fumigated. Our sources of water, creeks, rivers, lakes, have been poisoned, killing our fish and other living things …"∞

U.S. officials have said that large acreage of coca and poppy have been destroyed, "proving" that Plan Colombia has been successful, yet they have discouraged journalists from discussing the harmful effects of spraying Monsanto's chemicals. According to CorpWatch, a watchdog organization that investigates multinationals that profit out of war, fraud, environmental, and human-rights abuse, in January 2001 during a meeting with U.S. Embassy staff in Bogotá, the top officer at the State Department's Narcotics Affairs threatened CorpWatch by declaring, "You cannot mention Monsanto!"

CorpWatch said that when they requested more information about Monsanto and the program, a state-department official told the organization that the relationship between the U.S. government and Monsanto "is proprietary information between us and our supplier. It's exempt from the FOIA [Freedom of Information Act] requirements, too, so I don't think you will be able to get it."‡

Plan Colombia has not reduced the flow of cocaine to the U.S. but has alienated and destroyed the way of life for large numbers of Colombians. Thanks to U.S. taxpayers, Monsanto continues to profit while destroying indigenous peoples' health, food and water sources, and fish and wildlife.§

* † Brian Hansen. "Colombia: Monsanto, US War on Drugs Poison Environment." (November 20, 2000) Environment News Service. Source: CorpWatch. http://www.corpwatch.org/article.php?id=319

∞ ‡ Jeremy Bigwood. "Toxic Drift: Monsanto and the Drug War in Colombia." (June 21, 2001) CorpWatch. Source: Organic Consumers Association. www.organicconsumers.org/monsanto/toxicdrift.cfm

§ "Taxpayers Forced to Fund Monsanto's Poisoning of the Third World." Millions Against Monsanto. Source: Organic Consumers Association. www.organicconsumers.org/monlink.html

BIOTECH OPPRESSION

World Trade Organization Lawsuit

In other countries, genetic engineering has run into major obstacles: public opposition, grocery store owners removing GE foods from their shelves, third-world farmers resisting GE technology, and boycotts because GE foods have been labeled and consumers have the choice *not* to buy them.

Because of such opposition, biotech financial losses have been a concern to the industry and the U.S. government. As a result, some in the U.S. biotech industry—Monsanto, Aventis, DuPont, Dow Chemical—and big agricultural groups such as the National Corn Growers' Association lobbied the George W. Bush Administration to sue the EU because their regulatory system of GE foods had blocked millions of dollars of U.S. annual agricultural exports. In 2003, the U.S. government proceeded to file a complaint with the World Trade Organization (WTO) against the EU's de facto moratorium on GE food, as well as a number of EU member states' bans on GE food.

Greenpeace and other critics said the action was to discourage developing countries from implementing the 2003 Cartagena Protocol. The Cartagena Protocol on Biosafety is the first legally binding global agreement affirming the sovereign right of countries to reject or ban GE food on the basis of the Precautionary Principle. Therefore, according to Greenpeace, by attacking the

EU, the United States was warning developing countries not to use their rights under the Cartagena Protocol.[76]

As far as the WTO is concerned, laws and regulations of member countries need to be the least restrictive to trade as possible. Protecting food standards, the environment, and labor or human rights can be considered unnecessary restraints on trade. Furthermore, the WTO prohibits any government from discriminating against a product based on how it is made. To the WTO, food is food, whether it is organic, conventional, or genetically engineered.

In 2006, the WTO ruled that European safety bans on GE food is illegal under its global trade rules. Interestingly, the deputy director general of the WTO previously served as the European general counsel for Monsanto.

Regarding the EU, Greenpeace International trade advisor Daniel Mittler had this to say after the ruling:

> U.S. agro-chemical giants will not sell a bushel more of their GM grain as a result of the WTO ruling. European consumers, farmers, and a growing number of governments remain opposed to GMOs, and this will not change—in Europe or globally ... The U.S. administration and agro-chemical companies brought the case in a desperate attempt to force-feed markets with GMOs, but will continue to be frustrated ... [77]

Even though the WTO ruled in favor of the United States and biotechnology companies, Hungary declared that it is in its economic interests to remain GE-free, and Greece and Austria affirmed their total opposition to the crops. Italy has called the WTO ruling "unbalanced," and Poland's prime minister has pledged to keep the country GE-free. Local government is even more opposed: more than 3,500 elected councils in 170 regions of Europe have declared themselves GE-free.

According to the article *America's Masterplan is to Force GM Food on the World* by John Vidal in *The Guardian*, the reason the United States took Europe to the WTO court was to make it easier for its companies to open regulatory doors in China, India, Southeast Asia, Latin America and Africa, where most U.S. exports now go. This is where millions of tons of U.S. food aid is sent. More than two-thirds of exported U.S. corn goes to Asia and Africa, where once it went to Europe. India's largest farmers' organization said the result of the WTO verdict would be that the United States would become more aggressive in dumping GE food on developing countries.[78]

Anti-Labeling Campaigns

While awareness of and action against GE food remains strong in the EU and many other countries, most Americans remain uninformed or completely unaware. Since 1994, GE food has been force-fed to millions of American infants, children, and adults every day. Because the United States and Canada are the only industrialized countries in the world without a labeling law, most citizens do not even know they have been consuming GE food, which means they have not been able to make an informed choice not to eat it.

Unlike European countries and other nations where GE food is banned or labeled, food in the United States is not labeled if it contains GE ingredients. Most major U.S. food manufacturers do not avoid the use of GE ingredients in their products, but many of these same companies are GE-free in Europe: Coca-Cola, General Mills, Heinz, Hershey's, Kellogg's, Kraft, McDonald's, Burger King, Nabisco, Nestle, PepsiCo, Pillsbury, Procter & Gamble, Quaker Oats, and Safeway stores, just to name a few.[79]

In the United States in 2001, Rutgers University's Food Policy Institute conducted a four-year, $2.5 million study of consumer perceptions about food biotechnology. The results of the report, *Public Perceptions of Genetically Modified Foods: A National Study of American Knowledge and Opinion*, confirmed that an overwhelming majority, 94% of Americans, agreed that GE ingredients should be labeled.[80] The results of the study indicated that while most Americans know little about genetic engineering, many are uneasy about the potential long-term consequences of GE food or are at least willing to express some skepticism about its long-term safety.

The Genetically Engineered Foods Right to Know Act—a potential national labeling law—has been introduced by Ohio Representative Dennis Kucinich every year since 1999 and has never been voted on by Congress. Consumers in Europe and forty other countries have the right to know through labeling which foods contain GE ingredients, yet consumers in the United States, the home of freedom and democracy, continue to be denied this same right. In addition to attempts at a national labeling law, twenty-five pieces of legislation in fourteen states were introduced between 2001 and 2002 to call for either voluntary or mandatory labeling of all food products generated through biotechnology.[81] However, legislation requiring mandatory labeling of GE food has never passed.

One example of a proposed labeling initiative occurred in Oregon in 2002; it would have required the labeling of GE products in that state. Monsanto and other biotech companies, along with the food manufacturer industry, set a budget of $6 million to oppose the initiative based on the premise that "labeling would be cost-prohibitive to Oregonian consumers."[82] A Monsanto spokesperson said her company would support the anti-labeling campaign both through the anti-labeling Coalition Against the Costly Labeling Law and through biotech front group CropLife International. The coalition threatened that Oregonians would have to pay approximately $550 per family each year to have labeling regulations in place. Yet the pro-labeling side countered that countries with labeling laws have experienced minimal consumer costs due to regulation and labeling.

The anti-labeling (Monsanto-backed) coalition also claimed that the labeling plan was being "promoted by a small group of organic food companies that would benefit financially if consumers can be scared into buying their products."[83]

Mel Bankoff, founder of Emerald Valley Kitchen in Eugene, Oregon, who contributed $50,000 to the pro-labeling side of the campaign said, "I have to crack up when I hear them talk about me. I'm just a small food manufacturer who's concerned about this issue." He acknowledged the huge amounts of money that large corporations spent on the anti-labeling side.[84]

Supporters of labeling had a budget of roughly $150,000; it was no match for the $6 million public relations campaign of the biotech industry. The labeling initiative did not pass.

Preemption: "Monsanto" Laws in America

Some consumers and farmers have been trying to protect their local communities from the risks of GE crop contamination by passing local, city, and county ordinances to ban them. According to the June 2005 article *Ag Industry Aims to Strip Local Control of Food Supplies: Big Food Strikes Back* by Britt Bailey, founder and director of Environmental Commons, and Brian Tokar, who directs the Biotechnology Project at Vermont's Institute for Social Ecology,

> Since 2002, towns, cities, and counties across the United States have passed resolutions seeking to control the use of genetically modified organisms (GMOs) within their jurisdiction. Close to 100 New England towns have passed resolutions opposing the unregulated use of GMOs ... In 2004, three California counties, Mendocino, Trinity, and Marin, passed ordinances banning the raising of genetically engineered crops and livestock.

> Advocates across the country believe that the more people learn about the potential hazards of GE food and crops, the more they seek measures to protect public health, the environment, and family farms. They have come to view local action as a necessary antidote to inaction at the federal and state levels.[85]

In response, state legislators who support the biotech industry and food manufacturers have taken away the rights of cities and counties to ban GE crops. So far, fifteen states have passed preemption laws, or what have also been called "Monsanto Laws." In the past, state governments have overseen policies related to public health, safety, and welfare; yet no state regulates GE crops and livestock in a manner that protects public health and the environment. Biotech corporations have increasingly been trying to stop debate by eliminating local regulation of GE crops.[86]

Food Disparagement Laws

Food disparagement lawsuits can be brought on behalf of food products, forcing people to spend a lot of time and money in court if they question, without verifiable scientific proof, the safety of any food product. At least thirteen states have statutes that authorize lawsuits against anyone who "disparages" a food product; in addition, the Colorado legislature passed a criminal law designed to punish those found guilty of disparaging farm products.[87]

As Ronald K.L. Collins and Paul McMasters noted in their 1998 article *Veggie-Libel Law Still Poses a Threat* in *Legal Times*:

> Food disparagement laws encourage lawsuits designed to intimidate food critics by the mere threat of we-can-bankrupt-you litigation, replete with gag orders from cooperative judges ... As long as food critics must satisfy a high

burden of scientific proof, the media will be understandably hesitant to publish stories in this area lest their names be added to a legal complaint.[88]

David Bederman, associate professor of law at Emory University Law School in Atlanta, Georgia, said in the 1997 article *SLAPP Happy: Corporations That Sue to Shut You Up* by the Center for Media and Democracy's PR Watch.org,

> Agricultural disparagement statutes represent a legislative attempt to insulate an economic sector from criticism … as agricultural industries use previously untried methods as varied as exotic pesticides, growth hormones, radiation, and genetic engineering on our food supply. Scientists and consumer advocates must be able to express their legitimate concerns. The agricultural disparagement statutes quell just that type of speech … Any restriction on speech about the quality and safety of our food is dangerous, undemocratic, and unconstitutional.[89]

Genetic Pollution

For years, organic farmers have known that cross-pollination, or genetic pollution, of GE crops has the potential to contaminate their farms. By destroying farmers' organic status, it destroys their organic business.

Percy Schmeiser is a farmer from Saskatchewan, Canada, whose canola fields were contaminated with Monsanto's GE Roundup Ready canola by pollen from a nearby farm. Monsanto said it did not matter how the contamination took place and demanded Schmeiser pay Monsanto's technology fee. According to Schmeiser, "If I would go to St. Louis [Monsanto's U.S. headquarters] and contaminate their plots, destroy what they have worked on for forty years, I think I would be put in jail and the key thrown away."[90]

In 2002, Ontario farmer Alex Nurnberg had tests conducted on his one hundred-ton harvest of organic corn and found that twenty tons were contaminated. Nurnberg believed GE corn on a neighboring farm was the culprit. According to the Save Organic Food Web site, Terra Prima, an organic tortilla chips manufacturer, had to destroy eighty-seven thousand packages of corn chips when European importers discovered traces of GE corn in the chips. It was the first time a food manufacturer lost money due to genetic contamination.

Just as concerning is the fact that since 1991, the USDA has approved nearly four hundred field tests of crops that produce pharmaceuticals ("pharmacrops") and industrial compounds, which have also leaked into the food supply. In the twenty years since the USDA started to regulate field tests, it has approved nearly fifty thousand field sites. However, an internal audit commissioned by the USDA inspector general and released in December 2005 said the agency lacked basic information about test sites, failed to inspect field tests sufficiently, and neglected what happened to the crops after testing.[91, 92]

Regrettably, no amount of regulation can guarantee that GE crops will not contaminate non-GE crops. For plants pollinated by wind and insects, such as canola, pollen transfer is a constant threat. The British Soil Association's report *Seeds of Doubt* had this to say: "Widespread GM contamination has occurred rapidly and caused major disruption at all levels of the agricultural industry, for seed resources, crop production, food processing, and bulk commodity trading. It has undermined the viability of the whole North American farming industry.[93]

In response to the reality that contamination of non-GE crops by GE versions is inevitable, BIO and the U.S. grain industry requested in 2005 that the George W. Bush Administration expedite a policy governing contamination. Seven months after the request, the FDA submitted a document for publication in the *Federal Register* that would provide "safety assurance while recognizing a biological material's potential to appear in unexpected places as a result of biological factors ..."[94]

According to BIO's Web site, this "win" was the first step in formulating a global policy that recognizes inevitable contamination, which releases biotech companies from liability.

American Legislative Exchange Council

Just how do pro-industry, anti-democratic, anti-consumer-protection laws get their start? One way is through organizations like the American Legislative Exchange Council (ALEC). With annual revenues in excess of $5 million, ALEC advances the agendas of its corporate backers in state legislatures across the country.

As state governments have played a role in setting public policy, many of the nation's largest corporations and associations have invested millions of dollars into tax-exempt organizations that help them establish relationships with state lawmakers and executives. In exchange, such organizations provide corporate sponsors with access to elected officials and the opportunity to influence the policies recommended to state and local governments across the country. Most of the organizations are subsidized by taxpayer funds handed out by state legislature allowances, which fund a large share of their operating costs.[95]

ALEC is a membership organization consisting of nine task forces comprised of legislators and private industry representatives from across the United States. Its Natural Resources task force is devoted to biotechnology in agriculture. According to the ALEC Web site, its membership exceeds 2,400 state legislators from both political parties, which is 40% of the 7,500 state lawmakers in America. The group's corporate donors—some pay membership dues of $50,000 a year—have included Monsanto, DuPont, Enron, ExxonMobil, Philip Morris, and Chevron.

Members draft bills together, which are then introduced in state legislatures across the country. With funds coming from corporations and industry groups, members introduced more than 3,100 bills based on its models and passed 450 into law in 2000 alone. Most of the bills, of course, benefit the companies that helped write them.[96]

At a May 2004 meeting, industry groups proposed the "Biotechnology State Uniformity Resolution," which makes it illegal for communities to pass local protection laws against GE seeds, crops, or animals.[97] These preemption bills, also known as "Monsanto Laws," have been signed into law in Georgia, Michigan, Pennsylvania, Iowa, Idaho, North Dakota, South Dakota, Arizona, Oklahoma, Ohio, West Virginia, Texas, Kansas, Indiana, and Florida. They are working their way through legislatures in other states.[98]

Defenders of Wildlife and the Natural Resources Defense Council have been critical of ALEC because they say corporations can buy access to state legislatures, partly funded by taxpayers who, in many states, pay for legislators to attend ALEC meetings. In 2002, the organizations described ALEC as corrosive, secretive, highly influential, and a "tax-exempt screen for major U.S. corporations and trade associations that use it to influence legislative activities at the state level."[99]

A concern is that ALEC allows corporations to write public policy in secret. Brad DeVries of Defenders of Wildlife said, "It brings together some of the most powerful corporate interests to sit down and write legislation, which is then offered around the country without their fingerprints on it."[100]

In August 2005, President George W. Bush spoke at the Thirty-second Annual Meeting and praised ALEC for its results-oriented policies.

Chapter 4
Biotech Persuaders

In three investigations in 2005, Congress' Government Accountability Office (GAO) declared that government-made [video news releases] may constitute "covert propaganda" and said federal agencies may not produce news reports "that conceal or do not clearly identify for the television viewing audience that the agency was the source of those materials."

However, the Justice Department and the Office of Management and Budget instructed all executive branch agencies to ignore the GAO findings.[1]
David Barstow and Robin Stein's New York Times article "Under Bush, a New Age of Prepackaged Television News"

A children's propaganda piece, *Your World: Biotechnology and You,* funded by U.S. taxpayers and (among others) Monsanto, Pfizer, Novartis, Biotechnology Industry Organization, BioAlliance, and the Council for Biotechnology Information, has been distributed free to thousands of schools in the United States and Europe.

Touted as "educational materials, perfect for kindergarten through high school students," the goal is to support "science education and grassroots efforts that improve the understanding and acceptance of biotechnology."[2]
Susan Whitehead's Peace and Freedom article "New Biotech Propaganda Targets Children"

Why is it that most Americans, unlike people from other countries, have little or no idea they are eating GE food and that a major controversy exists over possible health hazards associated with it?

For years, the U.S. government and the biotech public relations industry's effort to "educate" journalists, politicians, and the public has enabled biotech food to be forced on an unsuspecting American public. In short, media coverage and propaganda promote the image of GE food as being harmless and necessary.

CENSORSHIP

Not unlike suppression in the scientific community, censorship in the media is widespread. The First Amendment right of freedom of the press should shed light on the truth and provide a level of checks and balances. Unfortunately, this right is dwindling due to corporate-owned media and the fear of lawsuits and job loss.

Fox TV

In 1996, Fox News in Tampa hired two investigative reporters, Steve Wilson and Jane Akre, to do a four-part series on Florida's milk and Monsanto's Posilac (rBGH). After researching the story for more than a year, Wilson and Akre reported about rBGH's harmful effects on human and cow health, as well as Monsanto's efforts to keep the truth suppressed. Monsanto learned about the report in advance and told Fox not to air the story. Monsanto's attorneys said Fox would suffer "enormous damage" if the report aired and warned of "dire consequences" for Fox News if they ran the story. As a result, the station canceled the story, and Fox executives asked Wilson and Akre to rewrite it.

According to the April 1998 article *Milk, rBGH, and Cancer* in *Rachel's Environment & Health Weekly*, Fox executives were not happy with any of the reporters' eighty-three revisions, so Fox wrote their own version of the original story, and among other changes, replaced the word "cancer" with "human health effects."[3] Wilson and Akre were offered financial compensation to keep quiet about the changes made to their report. They refused and countered with a lawsuit against the station in 1998, charging that Fox violated its license from the Federal Communications Commission by demanding that the reporters include false information in their story about Posilac.

In 2000, a Florida state court jury found Fox guilty of wrongful dismissal under Florida's whistleblower protection laws. However, according to the article *How Low Can Monsanto Go?* in *The Huffington Post*, Fox appealed, and in February 2003, a Florida Court of Appeals ruled in favor of Fox. The reason: there is no law against a news media outlet deliberately distorting and falsifying news. Therefore, if no laws were broken, the reporters were not considered whistleblowers. Apparently, Fox's defense rested on the premise that the First Amendment grants broadcasters the right to lie or deliberately distort news reports.[4]

Magazines Pulped

According to the *Z Magazine* article *The Ecologist and Monsanto,* in 1998, a small Cornwall-based company that had printed the British publication *The Ecologist* for twenty-six years decided to shred fourteen thousand copies of the 1998 September/October *Monsanto Files* issue of the magazine, apparently fearing legal action by Monsanto. The issue exposed Monsanto, including reviews of its corporate disasters involving Agent Orange, PCBs, rBGH, Roundup, and "terminator technology." It also included criticism from the Prince of Wales.

After the *Monsanto Files* issue was destroyed, the editors of *The Ecologist* had offers from other small printers in Britain who offered their services, assuring them that no threats from Monsanto would prevent them from publishing a document that "must be read by decision makers and the general public." A second batch of sixteen thousand copies was printed. The sixty-page exposé of Monsanto ended up being the best-selling issue of that magazine when four hundred thousand copies in a dozen languages were sold.[5]

BIOTECH FRONT GROUPS

In Sheldon Rampton's and John Stauber's book *Trust Us, We're Experts: How Industry Manipulates Science and Gambles with Your Future*, the authors state that people count on "experts" to tell them, for example, what is safe, what is nutritious, and what is scientifically "proven," because there is so much information available today and each person cannot be an expert in everything.

However, fabricating so-called "independent experts" by corporations and government occurs regularly without the public's awareness.[6] A front group is an organization that appears to represent one agenda while in reality it serves some other party or industry group whose sponsorship is usually concealed or rarely mentioned. If you ever want to know who is promoting a specific biotechnology "viewpoint," follow the money and find out which corporations fund the organization or individual.

Hudson Institute

The Hudson Institute is funded by many corporations; among them are Monsanto, Dow AgroSciences, DuPont, ConAgra, Cargill, and Novartis.

Dennis Avery is a senior fellow of the Hudson Institute and director of its Center for Global Food Issues (CGFI). He is also an advisor to the American Council on Science and Health and author of *Saving the Planet with Pesticides and Plastic*. Before joining Hudson, Avery served from 1980 to 1988 as the senior agricultural analyst for the U.S. State Department, where he was involved in assessing the foreign policy implications of food and farming developments.[7]

In 2005, when the Tillamook County Creamery Association in Oregon, the country's second-largest cheese producer, chose not to use Monsanto's Posilac on their dairy cows, the Hudson Institute attempted to discredit Tillamook. Hudson claimed that rBGH "doesn't change the milk a bit."[8] However, cancer researchers have discovered that elevated levels of IGF-1 in rBGH-injected cows may cause cancer in humans and that cows have mastitis and other health problems resulting from the synthetic hormone.[9, 10]

Hudson claimed that a report by the Physicians for Social Responsibility regarding cows having serious health problems were unfounded. But according to the report *Down on the Farm: The Real rBGH Story—Animal Health Problems, Financial Troubles*, details were revealed about catastrophic problems farmers encountered after trying rBGH. Sometimes these profound health problems with the cows led to the slaughter of their herds.[11]

In January 2006, Scripps Howard News Service announced it would terminate its relationship with columnist Michael Fumento, a senior fellow at the Hudson Institute. In his career with Hudson, Fumento has regularly opposed critics of the biotechnology industry in his column. It was discovered that Fumento received payments from Monsanto, the company that regularly was lauded in his opinion columns and in a book he wrote.[12]

CGFI is a project of the Hudson Institute with Dennis Avery as director. It, too, is an industry front group funded in part by Monsanto. In early 2005, CGFI launched a "Milk is Milk" campaign, claiming there is no difference between milk produced by cows injected with rBGH and organic milk.[13]

International Food Information Council

The International Food Information Council's (IFIC) mission is "to communicate science-based information on food safety and nutrition to health and nutrition professionals, educators, journalists, government officials and others providing information to consumers. IFIC is supported primarily by the broad-based food, beverage, and agricultural industries."[14] Some of the companies that fund IFIC are Monsanto, DuPont, Frito-Lay, Coca Cola, and Searle (a pharmaceutical division of Monsanto). Notably, a Monsanto representative is on IFIC's advisory board.[15]

In 1992, IFIC hired Dr. G. Clotaire Rapaille, an international market-research expert, to advise the biotech industry on ways to win public support for GE foods. IFIC wanted to know how it could overcome consumer concerns about the new technology, so a team consisting of representatives from Monsanto, NutraSweet, DuPont, Kraft, General Foods, and Calgene assisted in the research. The goal of the research team was to "develop actionable strategies, messages, and language that will express information positively about the process and products, without stirring fears or negative connotations."[16]

The suggested "words to lose" were scientific, such as DNA, gene-splicing, scientists, and genetically engineered, while many of the "words to use" were vague, emotional words designed to obscure the details about biotechnology, such as wholesome, natural order, cross-breeding, and genetically improved.[17]

The industry has increasingly replaced the terms "genetically modified organisms" and "genetically engineered" with "genetically improved foods" and "improved foods through biotechnology."

National Center for Food and Agricultural Policy

The National Center for Food and Agricultural Policy's (NCFAP) main biotechnology research program was launched in the spring of 2001 with financial support from Monsanto, the USDA, BIO, the biotech-industry funded Council for Biotechnology Information, and CropLife America.[18] The organization describes itself as "a private nonprofit non-advocacy research organization." However, NCFAP is a pro-GE industry group conducting studies in four areas: biotechnology, pesticides, international trade and development, and farm and food policy. NCFAP began to focus on GE crops in 2000.

In April 2004, NCFAP sponsored Greg Conko, of the lobby group the Competitive Enterprise Institute, to lobby farmers in the Australian states that were making decisions on possible large-scale GE trials being sought by Monsanto and Bayer.

The U.S. Embassy organized Conko's trip in an attempt to bolster waning interest in GE crops among Australian farmers.

CropLife America

CropLife America is a trade association representing the manufacturers of pesticides and other agricultural chemicals. It had been known as the American Crop Protection Association and prior to that was known as the National Agricultural Chemicals Association. "CropLife America member companies produce, sell, and distribute virtually all the crop protection and biotechnology products used by American farmers," says its Web site.[19]

In March 2004, CropLife America contributed more than $500,000—more than seven times that of the initiative supporters—to attempt to defeat the Mendocino county ballot initiative that would make the California county the first to ban GE crops. Despite the huge financial campaign against the initiative, Mendocino still passed the ban.

American Council on Science and Health

The American Council on Science and Health (ACSH) receives 76% of its funding from corporations and 17% of its funding from private foundations, according to Congressional Quarterly's Public Interest Profiles. The organization describes itself as "a consumer education consortium concerned with issues related to food, nutrition, chemicals, pharmaceuticals, lifestyle, the environment, and health."[20]

ACSH is heavily funded by corporations with direct interest in ACSH's chosen causes. Some current and past ACSH corporate and foundation funders are Monsanto, Kraft General Foods, Pfizer, Chevron, Coca-Cola, PepsiCo, Dow Chemical, Gerber, Hershey Foods, Merck Pharmaceutical, Shell Oil, Amoco, Exxon, Ford Motor Company, DuPont, and many more.[21]

Since it was established in 1978, the organization has defended the use of many food additives and chemicals that have been promoted by corporate interests. Monsanto and its subsidiaries, G.D. Searle and the NutraSweet Company, gave ACSH $105,000 in 1992, making Monsanto its "largest funder," according to an ACSH memo.[22]

Congress of Racial Equality

The Congress of Racial Equality (CORE) is an African-American group that played a leading role in the American civil-rights movement. During the late 1960s, however, CORE disassembled, and Roy Innis took over what remained. Today, the group has ties to Monsanto and has become an advocate for GE foods.

In January 2005, CORE organized two events for their Dr. Martin Luther King celebrations. One of these was a U.N. World Conference promoting GE foods, and the other was CORE's reception where they honored, among others, Karl Rove. Hugh Grant, chairman and CEO of Monsanto, was the chairman for the reception honoring Rove.

A little-known fact is that Monsanto is one of CORE's corporate partners.

In 2005, CORE produced a Monsanto-funded video called "Voice from Africa." The director and scriptwriter had worked on previous Monsanto projects. It was based on interviews with GE cotton farmers in South Africa, who were paid to claim sizeable benefits from Monsanto's GE cotton,[23] even though a five-year study showed that small-scale South African cotton farmers have not benefited from GE cotton.[24]

Competitive Enterprise Institute

The Competitive Enterprise Institute (CEI) is a nonprofit public-policy organization "dedicated to advancing the principles of free enterprise and limited government." CEI states on their Web site: "... overregulation of biotech foods harms consumers by denying them safer, less expensive, and more nutritious food choices."[25] The Washington front group has a multi-million dollar budget funded by major U.S. corporations such as Monsanto, Dow Chemical, Philip Morris, and Pfizer. In 2000, CEI had income of more than $3 million a year, with another million in assets.

Consumer Federation of America

Set up in 1968 to advocate consumer interests, the Consumer Federation of America (CFA) is also influenced by industry interests. The person in charge is Carol Tucker Foreman, who previously worked for the USDA and as a Monsanto lobbyist. She helped push rBGH into the American milk supply without labeling. Foreman did not support legislation that would require mandatory labeling, while other major consumer groups endorsed the legislation. Foreman, the "consumer" advocate, said when it comes to food risks that "the population tends to be extremely risk averse and not rational about food."[26]

At a conference on food policy sponsored by CFA in Washington, D.C. in 2000, most of the participants came from the agribusiness and biotech industries.

GOVERNMENT- AND INDUSTRY-SPONSORED PROPAGANDA

Government-Biotech Promotion

As part of a special taxpayer-funded project to promote GE crops worldwide, the U.S. State Department launched a Web site about biotech crops in 2004. *U.S. Regulatory Agencies Unified Biotechnology* resulted from the support initiative to "encourage broader adoption and acceptance of biotechnology in the developing world."[27] The Web site was developed with support from the Agricultural Biotechnology Support Fund, the USDA, FDA, and EPA.

The State Department's Biotechnology and Textile Trade Policy Division sends speakers around the world, funds workshops for "decision makers," and facilitates regulator-to-regulator meetings. National director of the Organic Consumers Association, Ronnie Cummins commented, "The State Department's promotion of an unpopular technology shows that these companies are having to turn to the Bush administration ... to basically force these crops on people.[28]

Video News Releases

A video news release (VNR) is a "fake news" video segment created by public relations firms, advertising agencies, marketing firms, corporations, and government agencies. Professional reporters are often used in VNRs, which can mislead the public into believing they are viewing real news stories. To unsuspecting viewers, VNRs, which typically do not disclose the source of the information, are little more than advertisements.

Corporations use public relations firms to produce VNRs that are then distributed to the media to inform, shape public opinion, promote commercial products, or for other interests. One of the largest distributors of VNRs is Medialink Worldwide, Inc. Fox TV has an arrangement with Medialink to distribute VNRs to 130 affiliates through its video-feed service called Fox News Edge. CNN distributes VNRs to 750 stations in the United States and Canada through CNN Newsource, and Associated Press Television News uses its Global Video Wire. It has been estimated that 90% of newsrooms today rely on VNRs.[29]

VNR use is not limited to corporations. They are also produced and distributed for the U.S. government by private contractors, the State Department's Office of Broadcasting Services, the USDA's Broadcast Media and Technology Center (BMTC), and the Defense Department's Pentagon Channel.

The USDA's BMTC offers full-service digital production facilities to USDA agencies, the White House, Departments of Energy, Defense, Housing and Human Services, Treasury, the U.S. Trade Representatives' Office, and the EPA. For the USDA alone, BMTC produces more than ninety VNRs and more than two thousand radio news stories, or audio news releases a year, in addition to public service announcements. The BMTC Web site says its VNRs cover "mission messages" in such areas as trade, biotechnology, small farms, and marketing.[30] These "news stories" are produced without any acknowledgement of the government's role in their production.[31]

With its $2.8 million annual budget, BMTC is, according to David Barstow and Robin Stein in the March 2005 *New York Times* exposé *Under Bush, a New Age of Prepackaged Television News*, "one of the most effective public relations operations inside the federal government."[32] The Bush Administration spent $254 million of taxpayer money in its first term on public relations contracts, more than double what the Clinton Administration spent in its second term.[33]

In three investigations in 2005, Congress' Government Accountability Office (GAO) declared that government-made VNRs may constitute "covert propaganda" and said federal agencies may not produce news reports "that conceal or do not clearly identify for the television viewing audience that the agency was the source of those materials."[34] However, the Justice Department and the Office of Management and Budget instructed all executive branch agencies to ignore the GAO findings.

America's Heartland—Brought to You by Monsanto

Monsanto and the American Farm Bureau Federation sponsored *America's Heartland*, a KVIE in Sacramento PBS television series, consisting of twenty half-hour episodes per year to run for two years. The idea for the show grew from *California's Heartland*, which ran successfully for seven years on PBS stations throughout the San Joaquin Valley. With major funding by Monsanto, *America's Heartland* was given the approval needed to go national in 2005.[35]

Proponents of the show said *America's Heartland* was intended to educate citizens about farming but critics believed it was to positively influence Americans' views toward factory farming and GE food.

Craig Culp, spokesperson for the Center for Food Safety said, "They [PBS] have an absolute obligation as stewards of public television to find underwriters for this series that do not include industries and organizations that can directly benefit from the airing of that program." Culp was critical of a 2002 *California Heartland* show on GE foods, saying it "was clearly developed to, if not actively promote GE foods and crops, certainly to place it in a favorable light, and put the opposition in a sort of negative or questionable light."[36]

In a letter sent to PBS managers about *America's Heartland*, seventy groups—including Institute for Agriculture and Trade Policy, Public Citizen, Friends of the Earth, and the Organic Consumers Association—suggested that stations should either drop the series or schedule complementary programming to expose *Heartland* as propaganda.

"The destruction of America's rural communities and the disappearance of its small farmers is an important story that needs to be told," the letter stated. "This story, one of rural depopulation, dwindling economic opportunities, industrial levels of pollution, and their attendant health and social concerns, is the ugly reality of the excesses that come from the unregulated large-scale industrialized agricultural system promoted by corporate America." [37] The critics said they were concerned that *America's Heartland* was being produced to project a positive image on the causes of these problems.

While the investment was significant for Monsanto, it was a clever public relations move. "We project that the first season of the program will be available in markets totaling more than 60% of the nation's viewers, approximately one hundred stations reaching more than 71 million households," said Jim O'Donnell, director of program marketing at KVIE in Sacramento.[38] A spokesperson for the American Farm Bureau Federation said, "We're after an urban audience and it's very hard to reach that audience with a traditional media. Public TV has a very respected brand and a very respected audience … That's one [agriculture] groups would be struggling to reach."[39]

Though the station has the right to choose which stories to use, it consults with a national advisory board that includes representatives from groups like the National Corn Growers Association, National Cattlemen's Beef Association, and the biotech industry-funded International Food Information Council.[40]

America's Heartland debuted in 2005, showcasing south Texas cattle ranching, locally grown crops, and research being conducted on a particular variety of GE sugarcane.[41]

Children and Biotech "Education"

The U.S. government and biotechnology companies want to make sure that the next generation is "educated" about biotech foods. Using taxpayer dollars along with corporate funds, "biotech education" publications have been disseminated to children in public schools.

The Agriculture in the Classroom (AITC) organization is a "grassroots program coordinated by the United States Department of Agriculture," designed "to help students gain a greater awareness of the role of agriculture ... so that they may become citizens who support wise agricultural policies," according to the AITC's Web site.[42] Individuals representing agribusiness, government, and education carry out the program in each state. Monsanto, an AITC partner, donated $50,000 to AITC to support "science education and grassroots efforts that improve the understanding and acceptance of biotechnology."[43] Some other AITC partners who make annual contributions include CropLife America, Altria (Kraft/Phillip Morris), IFIC, United Soybean Board, Fertilizer Institute, and the USDA.

The USDA supports the state groups by acting as a clearinghouse for materials and information while coordinating with national organizations to promote the goal of an increased awareness of agriculture among U.S. students.

One of the prominent industry-created materials is an ongoing children's magazine called *Your World: Biotechnology & You*, which, financially supported by U.S. taxpayers, has been distributed free to thousands of schools in the United States and Europe. *Your World* is sponsored by Monsanto, BIO, Pfizer, Novartis, Amgen, BioAlliance, Fischer Scientific, Genencor International, and the Council for Biotechnology Information.

According to the Biotechnology Institute's Web site, the organization is creating a base of understanding and awareness about biotechnology among teachers and students and is building the next generation of leaders in the industry. The Institute claims that each issue of *Your World* combines balanced, in-depth information on a feature topic and is an indispensable tool for bringing biotechnology into the classroom.

In the article *Weed Warriors: Herbicide Tolerant Crops* in the *Genetically Modified Food Crops* issue (volume 10, issue no. 1), Monsanto's Roundup is promoted to children as not being harmful to animals and as a safe alternative to other herbicides (it was stated that "glyphosate itself is less toxic than table salt"), even though Roundup has been linked to serious health effects, including cancer. In that same issue, an inset box titled "Organic Farming" states that many farms in the developing world are organic—not by choice, but because farmers have few resources. What do they tell children is the solution? "GM crops might be useful tools for them." On the last page of the publication (right next to the panel with sponsors' logos such as BIO, Monsanto Fund, Council for Biotechnology Information, Novartis, and others), children are assured that they "probably now understand more about these complex [biotech] issues than most adults" and are urged to "go and educate your elders!"[44]

Another industry children's publication, *Look Closer At Biotechnology*, is, according to the Council for Biotechnology Information's (CBI) Web site, a "fun and entertaining eighteen-page activity book incorporating short lessons, word puzzles, games, and quizzes to help children learn more about biotechnology." [45] Founded in 2000 by the biotech industry, CBI is an industry organization dedicated to promoting biotechnology in agriculture. Member companies and associations include Monsanto, BIO, DuPont, Dow, CropLife America, Bayer, and Syngenta. Biotech materials are touted as educational tools, perfect for kindergarten through high-school students.

Taxpayer-funded biotech "education" is abundant in schools today. How much taxpayer money goes into teaching children about alternative farming systems? Are children being presented biotech information to help them gain a greater awareness of the role of agriculture so that they may become citizens who support wise agricultural policies? Or is it so they will support biotech agricultural policies later on?

With a persistent corporate and government "spin" on biotech issues, the public is continuously uninformed and even misinformed. It is not surprising that Americans are unaware of the risks associated with GE food, particularly when the government and the biotech industry continue to use corporate and taxpayer funds to hide the truth, mislead, and at the very least, favorably influence public opinion about GE food through propaganda.

Chapter 5
Take It Personally

The evidence is clear and overwhelming: GE food is big business, purely and simply a profitable commodity to be bought and sold on the global market. The future of GE agriculture is unknown, but as a $6.15 billion industry in 2006, its growth and the corporate power behind it are undeniable.

Biotech proponents have said critics of GE food are anti-science, irrational, uninformed, and anti-technology. On the contrary, biotech critics have legitimate concerns and want more unbiased information to gain a science-based, rational policy on GE food. What is lacking is proof of its safety.

Why did the biotech industry and the government unleash GE food in America so quickly without public debate? Do you really believe if GE food were labeled it would "confuse" you, as has been claimed?

Agricultural biotechnology is not a precise science. There is no proof of safety and never has been. Consumers do not benefit from eating GE food, yet bear potential health risks. Why?

Until GE food has been *proven to be safe*, why should you be a guinea pig for the biotech industry? What if it were discovered that the GE food you're eating is *not* safe?

What can you do to safeguard yourself and your family?

In a Transgenic Nutshell

The biotech industry claims GE food is necessary to feed the world, but evidence suggests that the aim of the biotech industry is to help itself, not the poor. As a matter of fact, studies have shown that GE food has not been proven safe, does not feed the world, does not improve crop yields, does not require fewer pesticides, is not cost-effective for farmers, and is not rigorously regulated. Further, contamination of non-GE crops is an inevitable reality.

Conflicts of interest are pervasive in the scientific community today. Some scientists who have spoken out against GE foods have experienced censorship, while others who have discovered incriminating evidence or expressed concerns about biotechnology have been fired, threatened, and/or stripped of responsibilities. The potential impact of GE food on American public health, the environment, and the future is uncertain. Life does not get more personal than the food we eat every day. When some health problems, questionable results, or issues have surfaced or have been uncovered in laboratory animals after consuming GE food, they have not been appropriately investigated or researched further to protect human health.

Corporations have been permitted to keep undesirable GE test results out of public view by claiming "confidential business information," even when adverse health effects have been conclusive. Of the few relevant peer-reviewed safety tests on GE food, most have been conducted directly or under the auspices of the biotech industry, and many have been deemed scientifically flawed by independent scientists.

Governments in many other countries have banned GE food outright, or at least labeled it, giving their citizens a choice *not* to eat GE food. Americans know so little about GE food—or do not even know they are eating it—primarily because open, uncensored public discussion is extremely limited or non-existent, and because labeling of GE food in the United States is not required. Consumers in a democratic society have a right to truthful labeling in order to make informed choices for themselves and their families, even if labeling might be perceived as a "warning" to consumers not to eat them.

To provide a one-sided image of GE food as necessary and beneficial, propaganda in America has been disseminated via biotech front groups, government-

and industry-sponsored video news releases on television, audio news releases on the radio, Web sites, as well as government- and industry-sponsored children's biotech "education." At the same time, multi-million dollar anti-labeling campaigns and preemption laws have been passed to prevent local governments from banning GE food.

It is easy to see how unsuspecting consumers in America have been kept in the dark about GE food and why the biotech industry has grown significantly, even though evidence or scientific consensus that GE food is safe for human consumption has never been established. Americans are risking their health in return for non-existent and largely unproven consumer benefits; yet U.S. taxpayers unknowingly prop up the biotech industry and multinational corporate profits by massively funding GE crop and dairy subsidies, state initiatives, tax breaks, foreign aid, and other biotech support doled out by the U.S. government.

TAKE ACTION

Despite what first may appear to be insurmountable obstacles, you can still make informed food choices and avoid GE food. You can make your voice heard through your purchasing decisions and dollars spent.

The first step is to realize that genetically altered food is an attack on your health freedom every time you eat. *It is personal.* Second, become informed and look for the truth. Look beyond the propaganda of the U.S. government, multinational corporations, and their front groups.

In short, until it is proven safe, you are eating GE food at your own risk. If you choose to stop being force-fed this untested, unlabeled food, you can take action now to protect yourself and your family. This is too important to put off until later—do something about it today.

Avoid GE Foods

Currently, the most common commercialized GE food in the United States includes non-organic soy, corn, canola, cotton, and dairy products. As a starting point, either eliminate them from your diet or buy organic equivalents. Remember that all of these foods exist in the American food supply, most often in their various derivative forms in processed foods. For example, soy ingredients such as lecithin, soy oil, and soy protein are found in 60-70% of all processed foods.

The True Food Now Network, a grassroots network of the Center for Food Safety, compiled a detailed 36-page shopping guide at www.truefoodnow.org/shoppersguide, focusing on foods items made with ingredients that are commonly genetically engineered.

Following are some of the most common GE ingredients and products to avoid:[1]

Soy

Soy flour, soy oil, soy lecithin, TVP, soy protein isolates and concentrates. Products that may contain GE soy derivatives are vitamin E, tofu dogs, cereals, vegetable burgers and sausages, tamari, soy sauce, chips, ice cream, frozen yogurt, infant formula, sauces, protein powder, margarine, mayonnaise, soy cheeses, crackers, breads, cookies, chocolates, candy, fried foods, shampoo, bubble bath, cosmetics, enriched flours, breads, and pastas.

Corn

Corn flour, cornstarch, corn oil, cornmeal, corn sweeteners, corn syrups, dextrose, maltodextrin, fructose, citric acid, and lactic acid. Products that may contain GE corn derivatives include vitamin C, tofu dogs, chips, candy, ice cream, infant formula, salad dressings, tomato sauces, breads, cookies, cereals, baking powder, alcohol, vanilla, margarine, soy sauce, tamari, soda, fried foods, powdered sugar, enriched flours, and pastas.

Canola

Oil. GE canola derivatives may exist in chips, salad dressings, cookies, margarine, soaps, detergents, soy cheeses, and fried foods. Canola oil is frequently used in restaurants.

Cotton

Cottonseed oil, fabric. Products that may contain GE cotton or its derivatives are clothes, linens, chips, peanut butter, crackers, and cookies.

Dairy Products

Milk, cheese, butter, buttermilk, sour cream, yogurt, whey. The questions to ask: Have the cows been treated with rBGH? What kind of feed have they been given? If they are not being fed organic grains, chances are that they eat GE animal feed. What does this do to their milk products?

Animal Products

Because animal feed is often genetically engineered, all animal products and byproducts are affected. Meat, eggs, and dairy products from animals that have eaten GE feed are questionable. Recently, the USDA has said milk and meat from cloned (GE) animals is "safe" for public consumption.

Other

Vitamins, papaya, food additives, enzymes, flavorings, and processing agents, including the sweetener aspartame, and rennet that is used to make hard cheeses.

Go Organic

Considering that the majority of conventional food products on the market have some GE ingredients in them, eating organic food is your best bet to avoid them. When you buy organic, no animals (except dairy cows prior to being moved to organic farms) are permitted to have been given antibiotics, growth hormones, or feed made from animal byproducts. No GE ingredients, irradiated ingredients, synthetic ingredients (pesticides, herbicides, etc.), or fertilizers made with sewage sludge are legally allowed in organic food. All of these are permitted in most conventional food production.

When you see a package labeled organic, but not "100%" organic, look at the ingredients closely. Be sure the non-organic ingredients are not the common GE ingredients such as soy, corn, canola, cottonseed oil, or dairy. Specifically look for packages labeled "GE-free, "rBGH-free," "Non-GMO," "No GMOs," "No bioengineered ingredients," and "Made with no genetically engineered ingredients."

When shopping, look at produce stickers; they have code numbers on them, depending on whether the item has been conventionally grown, organically grown, or genetically engineered. The code for conventionally grown produce begins with the number 4, organically grown produce begins with the number 9, and GE produce begins with the number 8. However, because GE food is considered the same as conventional by the FDA, you probably won't find a number-8 sticker in U.S. grocery stores.

Organic food can cost more than conventional food, primarily because small organic farms produce more labor-intensive products and do not qualify for government subsidies that large factory farms receive. To reduce your costs, comparison shop just as you would with conventional foods. Find out which stores have the lowest organic food prices and check out local farmer's markets, which can often be lower in cost. Farmer's markets listed by states can be found online at www.ams.usda.gov/farmersmarkets/map/htm.

See if there is a community-supported organic farm, community sustainable agriculture (CSA) co-op, or other local co-op near you. The savings can be considerable if you shop around.

Vote with your dollars—do not support companies that use GE ingredients or violate organic standards.

Let Your Opinion Be Known

Food Manufacturers and Restaurants

E-mail or write food manufacturers to let them know that, unless they go GE-free, you will stop buying their products. In restaurants, tell the owner or manager that you are concerned about GE foods and ask where they source their ingredients.

GE-Free Children's School Meals

According to Jeffrey M. Smith, director of the Institute for Responsible Technology and author of *Seeds of Deception* and *Genetic Roulette*, schools throughout the UK and parts of Europe banned GE food years ago. In the 1990s many Parent and Teacher Associations in the United States rallied against rBGH, and more than a hundred school districts banned milk from rBGH-treated cows.

Smith's DVD/VHS, *Hidden Dangers in Kids' Meals*, reveals that children face the greatest risk from the potential dangers of GE foods, mainly because young, fast-developing bodies are influenced most and because children are more susceptible to allergies, problems with milk, and nutritional problems.

The Institute for Responsible Technology supports efforts to create GE-free schools by providing written and audio-visual materials, Web support, and guidance to local campaigns. With support from the Sierra Club and others, the Institute for Responsible Technology makes available one or more copies of the *Hidden Dangers in Kids' Meals* video (DVD/VHS) and the CD *You're Eating WHAT?* to individuals or groups who are committed to starting a local GE-free school campaign or already have an existing campaign. Check out Smith's Web site at www.gmfreeschools.org.

Affect Legislation

Until they have been thoroughly tested and found safe for human health, any foods that contain GE ingredients should be labeled as such.

Get behind the Genetically Engineered Food Right to Know Act. The national bill introduced by Ohio Representative Dennis Kucinich would require food containing GE material to be labeled. Unfortunately, it has never reached the floor of either house of Congress, having been shelved in House committees since its introduction in 1999.

Senator Barbara Boxer also introduced the *Genetically Engineered Food Right to Know Act* in 2000, and stated, "Given the rapid expansion of this largely untested technology, we should provide consumers with the right to know whether they are eating genetically engineered food. Congress has already provided consumers similar rights by requiring the labeling of foods containing artificial colors and flavors, chemical preservatives, and artificial sweeteners." She commented that the United States has agreed to label its international shipments of seeds, grains, and plants that may contain genetically engineered material as part of a 131-nation trade agreement. "If we can provide this information to our trading partners, shouldn't we make similar information available to American consumers?"[2]

Let your senators and representatives know you want this law passed. If you do not know who they are, their contact information is available on The Campaign's Web site at www.thecampaign.org.

Add Your Voice to Organized Efforts

Bioneers Conference

Founded in 1990, Bioneers promotes practical environmental solutions and innovative social strategies for restoring the earth and communities. According to its Web site, Bioneers is a gathering of scientific and social innovators who have demonstrated visionary and practical models for restoring the earth and communities. It was created to conduct programs in the conservation of biological and cultural diversity, traditional farming practices, and environmental restoration.

In 2007, the conference was held in San Rafael, California. Beaming Bioneers combines a live satellite broadcast of the conference to various locations around the country with local workshops and activities geared toward specific regions. For more information, go to www.bioneers.org.

BioREALITY Conference

In 2007, The Campaign to Label Genetically Engineered Food held the first annual BioREALITY conference in Washington, D.C. It helped to fill a void in the effort to label and regulate GE food in the United States. The Campaign's proactive conference is to be held annually each spring. Visit www.bioreality.org or The Campaign at www.thecampaign.org for more information.

JIGMO—Joint International GM Opposition

When the deputy director general of the WTO, who previously served as the European general counsel for Monsanto, ruled in favor of GE crop producers against the European Union, critics were concerned that the GMO ruling would open the doors to the development of more GE crops, as well as the contamination of both GE-free fields and food chains.

As a result, 110 international organizations from more than fifty countries announced that April 8, 2006, would be "Joint International GM Opposition Day." The day featured public events in several countries to demonstrate continuing global opposition to GE foods and crops. A U.S. event promoter commented, "We will join with our allies around the world to condemn the WTO decision and to denounce the U.S. administration's attempts to impose this hazardous technology on us all."[3]

"The more people learn about the hazards of GMOs for our health, the environment, and traditional agricultural communities, the more they oppose this technology," said Brian Tokar of the Institute for Social Ecology in the United States. "And in many countries, this concern has been translated into sound public policies to limit the importation and growing of GE products. That is why corporations work to suppress public awareness in the U.S. and why our government has pressed the WTO to overrule sound protective actions in other countries."[4]

The event was such a success that the JIGMOD (Joint International GM Opposition Day) evolved into the Joint Actions of Information of GMOs, a month-long annual event in countries such as Malaysia, Japan, France, the United States, Turkey, Mexico, Belgium, and others. Visit http:// altercampagne.free.fr/ for more information.

Encourage GMO Contamination Testing

The Non-GMO Project

The Non-GMO Project grew out of the realization of natural and organic food retailers that they have a responsibility to give their customers informed choices and reliable access to non-GE products. As of 2007, the Project makes available to customers products that meet a credible and consistent non-GMO standard. While the U.S. National Organic Standards and the National Standard of Canada for Organic Agriculture assure that food and supplement ingredients carrying their organic label are not grown from GE seeds, neither program deals with the issues of genetic contamination.

The Non-GMO Project was founded by two natural grocery stores, The Natural Grocery Company in Berkeley, California, and The Big Carrot Natural

Food Market in Toronto, Canada. The Project has created a systematic and scientific program for non-GMO certification and has retained Genetic ID North America, the world's leader in GMO control and identification, to analyze and certify their products.

In a March 2007 press release, Straus Family Creamery said they will verify that all of their products are not contaminated by previously undetected GMOs. "Certified organic crops are at risk of contamination by genetically modified crops," said Albert Straus, President of Straus Family Creamery. "We have rejected organic feeds for our animals because of GMO contamination. We need better controls over our feeds and ingredients, so we have established this relationship with The Non-GMO Project to ensure that all of our products are verified as non-GMO."[5]

Whole Foods Markets, Inc., and United Natural Foods, Inc. also claimed in March 2007 that they will test their private-label organic and natural food lines to ensure products contain no GMOs through the Non-GMO Project. Likewise, Eden Foods and Lundberg Family Farms also announced their products will be tested as well.

Companies passing the verification process will bear the nonprofit's verification and compliance seal on product labels. "This program will function as an additional quality-assurance program for our customers," said Albert Straus of Straus Family Creamery. "The integrity of the organic movement cannot be damaged by the presence of GMOs."[6]

The Non-GMO Project is a nonprofit organization. Tell your local grocery store about them, ask store managers if they will join this effort, and let them know that you care about the presence of GMOs in our food supply. Contact www.nongmoproject.org.

THE FUTURE

Perhaps because the food supply is such a personal matter, many individuals and organizations are focused on shedding light on the concerns of GE food. Fortunately for the public, these combined efforts have raised awareness and united people on a worldwide level, thereby spawning new movements in agricultural sustainability, in responsibility for local self-subsistence, and in support of a return to small-scale farming practices that benefit their own communities—away from massive monoculture and destructive agribusinesses. Ultimately, each individual plays a pivotal role in this evolution and in the future.

Organic Agriculture and Food Security

Organic food—food grown and processed without chemicals, additives, hormones, or pesticides and without the use of genetic engineering—is being grown in more than 120 countries. Between 2002 and 2005 world sales of organic food increased by 43% from $23 billion to $33 billion and it is predicted that sales in 2006 will have reached $40 billion.[7]

The report *The World of Organic Agriculture, Statistics and Emerging Trends 2007* revealed that Australia has the greatest area of organically farmed land with approximately 11.8 million hectares (29.16 million acres), followed by Argentina with 3.1 million hectares (7.66 million acres), and China with 2.3 million hectares (5.68 million acres). The United States lags behind with only 1.6 million hectares (3.95 million acres),[8] even though North America is the largest market for organics.

While so much U.S. taxpayer funding goes into biotechnology R&D, why isn't more research going into organic farming? Could it be that multinational corporations cannot hugely profit from organic food, as they can with their GE crops using their proprietary seed-and-chemical-based systems?

A misconception exists that organic food cannot contribute to the global food supply due to low yields. That, however, has been shown to be untrue. Researchers from the University of Michigan found that organic farming can yield up to three times as much food on individual farms in developing countries, which refutes the claim that organic farming methods cannot produce enough food to feed the global population. "In developing countries, food production could double or triple using organic methods," said Ivette Perfecto, professor at the University of Michigan's School of Natural Resources and Environment, and one the study's principle researchers. "My hope is that we can finally put a nail in the coffin of the idea that you can't produce enough food through organic agriculture."[9]

According to the University of Michigan's July 2007 press release *Organic Farming Can Feed the Word, U-M Study Shows,* it was estimated that organic methods could produce enough food on a global per capita basis to sustain the current human population, and an even larger population, without increasing the land needed to grow food. In addition to high yields, researchers found those yields could be accomplished using existing quantities of organic fertilizers, which would reduce the detrimental environmental impacts of conventional agriculture's fertilizer runoff—the primary cause in creating dead zones, or low oxygen areas where marine life cannot survive.

Perfecto said the idea that people would go hungry with organic farming is ridiculous. "Corporate interest in agriculture and the way agriculture research has been conducted in land grant institutions, with a lot of influence by the chemical companies and pesticide companies as well as fertilizer companies—all have been playing an important role in convincing the public that you need to have these inputs to produce food."[10]

The international umbrella organization of worldwide organic agricultural movements, the International Fund for Agricultural Development (IFAD), sponsored an event in 2006 at a meeting of the United Nations Food and Agricultural Organization's (FAO) Committee on World Food Security, which has also drawn attention to the potential of organic agriculture for achieving global food security.

The IFAD presented evidence of the impact of organic agriculture on rural development and poverty alleviation. Organic farming is being recognized as a promising alternative for small farmers, who in most cases can easily shift to organic production. According to the assistant director-general of FAO, many countries want information on organic agriculture and its contribution to food security. Therefore, the FAO plans to hold an international conference on Organic Agriculture and Food Security in 2007; the resulting report will be submitted to the Committee on World Food Security.[11]

Replenish the Soil with Effective Microorganisms

The majority of GE crops today have been altered to tolerate massive doses of pesticides and herbicides or to create a pesticide in each of its cells. The transition from chemical-based farming systems (whether crops are GE or conventional) to a more sustainable agriculture will depend largely on what farmers do to improve and maintain the quality of their agricultural soils. Once that the transition from conventional agriculture to organic farming has occurred, farmers have found their new farming systems to be stable, productive, manageable, and profitable—without using chemical pesticides or GE crops.

Effective Microorganisms, called EM technology, is a method to improve soil quality and plant growth using a mixture of beneficial microorganisms. The concept of EMs was developed by Japanese agronomist Teruo Higa from the University of Ryukyus in Japan. He believes that a combination of approximately eighty different microorganisms is capable to influence decomposing organic matter so that it reverts into a "life-promoting" process.

EM technology may be a valuable resource to help farmers develop systems that are economically, environmentally, and socially sustainable. Higa claims that there are three groups of microorganisms: positive microorganisms for regeneration, negative microorganisms for decomposition and degeneration, and opportunist microorganisms.[12] Higa believes opportunist microorganisms will follow the trend of whichever microorganism is dominant for regeneration or degeneration; therefore, it is possible to affect the soil positively by supplementing positive microorganisms.

The misuse and excessive use of chemical fertilizers and pesticides has often adversely affected the environment and created many food safety and human and animal health problems. We do not know what will happen with the soil after GE crops have been planted and harvested year after year. At the same time, a growing interest has sprung forth in natural farming and organic agriculture by consumers and environmentalists as possible alternatives to chemical-based agriculture.[13] EM technology may be a means of favorably countering and revitalizing the soil from the yet unknown effects of GE agriculture.

GEAN's Four Core Principles for GE Food

According to their Web site, the Genetic Engineering Action Network (GEAN) seeks to support and further the work of those organizations and individuals working to address the risks to the environment, biodiversity, and human health, as well as the socioeconomic and ethical consequences of genetic engineering. GEAN is a network of almost one hundred organizations across the United States working to resist genetic engineering in agriculture. The organization offers four core principles necessary for the responsible use of GMOs:[14]

Choice

Prior informed choice is essential to a democratic and accountable food system. Therefore, the mandatory, clear, accurate, complete labeling of all products, whether foreign or domestic, derived from, processed with, produced by, containing or consisting of GE organisms should be required.

Assessment

A publicly enforced and fully transparent government system is needed to assess the socioeconomic, environmental, and human health impacts of genetic engineering that conforms to rigorous scientific standards, requires a demonstration of a reasonable certainty of no harm, shifts the burden of proof and cost to the manufacturer, and permanently codifies the Precautionary Principle.

Protection

Protecting family farmers, workers, consumers, and the environment is necessary to end all monopoly practices of corporate agribusiness by enforcing anti-trust and market concentration laws, banning patents of seeds, plants, animals, and terminator-type technologies, and renewing public interest agricultural research.

Liability

Any entity, excluding family farmers, engaging in research, development, or manufacturing of GE or modified products must assume all liability for harm to health and the environment, including, but not limited to the transfer of GE traits, transgenic drift, destruction of wildlife and habitat, and the short- and long-term effects on human health and the environment.

Resources

WEB SITES

Food Information and Organizations

Bioneers: *www.bioneers.org*

Bioneers was created to conduct programs (Beaming Bioneers, radio series, Bioneers buzz, Bioneers Youth Initiative) in the conservation of biological and cultural diversity, traditional farming practices, and environmental restoration. Their vision of environment encompasses the natural landscape, cultivated landscape, biodiversity, cultural diversity, watersheds, community economics, and spirituality. Bioneers seeks to unite nature, culture, and spirit in an earth-honoring vision and create economic models founded in social justice.

The Campaign to Label Genetically Engineered Food: *www.thecampaign.org*

The Campaign to Label Genetically Engineered Food is a nonprofit political advocacy organization started in 1999 "to create a national grassroots consumer campaign for the purpose of lobbying Congress and the President to pass legislation that will require the labeling of genetically engineered foods in the United States." In July 1999, The Campaign's executive director, Craig Winters, flew to Washington, D.C., to meet with Ohio Congressman Dennis Kucinich, who subsequently agreed to become the primary sponsor of legislation to label genetically engineered foods.

Letters can be found on their Web site, along with many other activist and educational tools. They encourage all concerned citizens to purchase copies of The Campaign's Take Action packets to share with friends and associates. Subscribe to their e-news alerts through their Web site.

111

Center for Food Safety: *www.centerforfoodsafety.org*

The Center for Food Safety (CFS) is a nonprofit public interest and environmental advocacy membership organization with the purpose of challenging harmful food production technologies and promoting sustainable alternatives. CFS combines multiple tools and strategies in pursuing its goals, including litigation and legal petitions for rulemaking, legal support for various sustainable agriculture and food safety constituencies, as well as public education, grassroots organizing, and media outreach.

Environmental Commons: *www.environmentalcommons.org*

Environmental Commons brings democracy and science to environmental decision-making at the local, state and national levels. They encourage involvement in the democratic process to defend our environmental heritage—water, air, biodiversity, and genetic variability, known as "the commons." According to director Britt Bailey, conserving the commons is linked to the quality of our lives: our health and the health of ecosystems. Environmental Commons also works to preserve natural areas, to protect wildlife, and to promote sustainable policies using education and informed discussion.

Environmental Commons believes that genetic modification and engineering constrict farmer seed and variety privileges, confer private ownership of otherwise commonly held life forms, create unanticipated environmental effects, threaten human health, suppress the development and integrity of less intensive, more sustainable farming systems, and damage local farming economies.

The Web site has news articles, reports, fact sheets, a food democracy legislation tracker, and more.

Friends of the Earth International: *www.foei.org*

With one million members and supporters around the world, Friends of the Earth International (FOEI) campaigns on today's urgent environmental and social issues. They challenge the current model of economic and corporate globalization, and promote solutions that will help to create environmentally sustainable and socially just societies.

According to their Web site, core themes running through the organization's work are "protecting human and environmental rights, protecting the planet's disappearing biodiversity, and the repayment of ecological debt owed by rich countries to those they have exploited for their own economic benefit." Specific campaigns include GE food, climate change, corporate accountability, fair trade, and others.

Genetic Engineering Action Network: *www.geaction.org*

Genetic Engineering Action Network (GEAN) is comprised of almost one hundred organizations across the United States working to resist genetic engineering in agriculture. The GEAN's affiliate groups range from large national nonprofits, including the Center for Food Safety and Friends of the Earth, to state and regional groups like Californians for GE-Free Agriculture and GMO-Free Hawaii, to small grassroots groups, like Colorado GEAN and GE-Free Maine. Their affiliates work on a variety of issues, including passing town- and county-level restrictions on GMOs, stopping the introduction of new GE crops, and advocating for tighter national and international standards on GMOs. They provide their affiliate groups with a wide range of support: they run a large listserv that connects activists from across the United States, they organize national and regional conferences for genetic-engineering activists, and they provide materials, strategy advice, media support, and trainings for emerging grassroots campaigns.

GM Watch: *www.gmwatch.org*

GM Watch has a global focus but developed as a news and research service founded in the UK to report on the growing concerns about genetic engineering. It focuses on the use of hype, propaganda, and spin to promote this technology and on exposing the role played by corporate-friendly scientists, industry front groups, public relations companies, lobbyists, and political groups.

GRAIN: *www.grain.org*

GRAIN is an international non-governmental organization that promotes the sustainable management and use of agricultural biodiversity based on people's control over genetic resources and local knowledge. It was established at the beginning of the 1990s to launch a decade of popular action against one of the most pervasive threats to world food security: genetic erosion. The loss of biological diversity undermines the very sense of "sustainable development," as it destroys options for the future and robs people of a key resource-base for survival. Central to their approach is that the conservation and use of genetic resources is too important to leave to scientists, governments, and industry alone. What started as a small Euro-centered organization in the early 1990s has grown into an organization with staff in nine countries across five continents, carrying out a broad and challenging program on local and global management of genetic diversity and the impacts of biotechnology on world agriculture, particularly in developing countries.

GRAIN produces several briefings each year. These are substantial research reports, providing in-depth background information and analysis on a give topic. *Against the Grain* is a series of short opinion pieces on recent trends and developments in the issues that GRAIN works on. Each one focuses on a specific and timely topic. *Seedling* is their quarterly magazine and flagship publication.

Institute for Agriculture and Trade Policy: www.iatp.org

The Institute for Agriculture and Trade Policy's (IATP) mission is to "promote resilient family farms, rural communities and ecosystems around the world through research and education, science and technology, and advocacy."

According to their Web site, in the 1980s, family farmers were told they were inefficient and they had to either get big or get out; an effort to save the family farm helped create the IATP. In 1986, the organization began documenting the underlying causes of America's rural crisis and proposing policies that would benefit farmers, consumers, rural communities, and the environment.

IATP works on several fronts: how global trade agreements impact domestic farm and food policies; alternative economic models that include clean sources of energy to stimulate rural development; sustainable forest management; how to stop the overuse of antibiotics in agriculture and aquaculture, while limiting the release of mercury and other toxic pollutants that fall onto farmland and enter the food supply; and the impact of GE crops on the environment, human health, and farmers' income.

Institute for Responsible Technology: www.responsibletechnology.org

Jeffrey M. Smith has counseled world leaders from every continent, influenced the first state laws regulating GMOs, and has united leaders to support *The Campaign for Healthier Eating in America*, a revolutionary industry and consumer movement to remove GMOs from the natural food industry. He has lectured in twenty-five countries and has been quoted by government leaders and hundreds of media outlets across the globe. Smith directs the *Campaign for Healthier Eating in America* from the Institute for Responsible Technology, where he is executive director. He wrote international bestseller *Seeds of Deception* and is the producer of the documentary video series, *The GMO Trilogy*. He writes an internationally syndicated monthly column, *Spilling the Beans*.

The Institute for Responsible Technology is a public-education nonprofit that works on major public initiatives with scientists and concerned citizens from around the world to shine a spotlight on the dangers of GMOs. Smith's priority program is GE foods and crops, seeking to ban the genetic engineering of the food supply and all outdoor releases of genetically modified organisms, at least until there is a consensus of scientific opinion that such products are safe and appropriate based on independent and reliable data. You can subscribe to his *Spilling the Beans* monthly free e-newsletter via www.responsibletechnology.org.

Natural Solutions Foundation: www.healthfreedomusa.org

The Natural Solutions Foundation (NSF) is a nonprofit organization devoted to protecting and promoting health freedom for all Americans. According to their Web site, "We know that alone we cannot safeguard our health freedoms. Therefore, the Natural Solutions Foundation is a 'network of networks' created to disseminate the facts, challenges, and triumphs in our shared battle to protect, preserve, and defend our right to make our own health choices based on what we, not the government, believe are the best choices for ourselves."

The NSF was created to protect, promote, and defend health freedom when Rima E. Laibow, M.D., and Major General Albert Stubblebine III (U.S. Army, Ret.) took stock of the "dismal state of health freedom in the United States." It is based on the belief that decisions that impact Americans' lives must be made through a democratic process in which their voices are heard and counted. Subscribe to NSF's free e-newsletter through the Web site.

Organic Consumers Association: www.organicconsumers.org

The Organic Consumers Association (OCA) is a complete resource, an online and grassroots nonprofit public interest organization campaigning for health, justice, and sustainability. The OCA focuses on crucial issues of food safety, industrial agriculture, genetic engineering, children's health, corporate accountability, fair trade, environmental sustainability, and other key topics. According to their Web site, they are the only organization in the United States focused exclusively on promoting the views and interests of the nation's estimated fifty million organic and socially responsible consumers. The OCA represents over 850,000 members, subscribers and volunteers.

The OCA was formed in 1998 due to the backlash by organic consumers against the USDA's controversial proposed dilution of the national regulations for organic food. Through the OCA's "Safeguard Organic Standards" campaign, the organic community has been able to mobilize hundreds of thousands of consumers to pressure the USDA and organic companies to preserve strict organic standards. The OCA also works with public interest groups to challenge industrial agriculture and the corporate globalization of the economy.

True Food Now: www.truefoodnow.org

The True Food Network is now the grassroots network of the Center for Food Safety. Established in 2000 as a way to engage non-farmers in the struggle against GE crops, the True Food Network is a member network dedicated to stopping the genetic engineering of food, farms, and future, and to working with others to create a socially just, democratic, and sustainable food system.

Science News

Center for Public Integrity: www.publicintegrity.org

The Center for Public Integrity is a nonprofit, nonpartisan, non-advocacy, independent journalism organization based in Washington, D.C., whose mission is to produce original investigative journalism about significant public issues to make institutional power more transparent and accountable. It generates accessible investigative reports, databases, and contextual analyses on issues of public importance and disseminates work to journalists, policymakers, scholars, and citizens using a combination of digital, electronic, and print media.

Center for Science in the Public Interest: *www.cspinet.org*

The Center for Science in the Public Interest is a consumer advocacy organization whose missions are to conduct innovative research and advocacy programs in health and nutrition and to provide consumers with current, useful information about their health and well-being. Its goals are to provide useful, objective information to the public and policymakers and to conduct research on food, alcohol, health, the environment, and other issues related to science and technology; to represent the citizens' interests before regulatory, judicial, and legislative bodies; and to ensure that science and technology are used for the public good and to encourage scientists to engage in public-interest activities.

Institute of Science in Society: *www.i-sis.org.uk*

The Institute of Science in Society (ISIS) is a not-for-profit organization founded in 1999 by Mae-Wan Ho and Peter Saunders to work for social responsibility and sustainable approaches in science. A major part of its work is to promote critical public understanding of science and to engage both scientists and the public in open debate and discussion. ISIS has been providing inputs into the GE debate that would have been lacking otherwise.

Union of Concerned Scientists: *www.ucsusa.org*

According to its Web site, the Union of Concerned Scientists (UCS) is the leading science-based nonprofit organization working for a healthy environment and a safer world. UCS combines independent scientific research and citizen action to develop innovative, practical solutions and to secure responsible changes in government policy, corporate practices, and consumer choices. The UCS is a reliable source for independent scientific analysis, with their scientists and policy experts frequently called to testify before government committees.

News and Other Information

Alliance for Bio-Integrity: ___www.biointegrity.org___

The Alliance for Bio-Integrity is a nonprofit, nonpolitical organization dedicated to the advancement of human and environmental health through sustainable and safe technologies. The Alliance's initial project is to gain a rational and prudent policy on GE food. This entails educating the public about the unprecedented dangers to the environment and human health posed by the massive enterprise to genetically reprogram the world's food supply; securing a scientifically sound system for safety-testing genetically altered foods; and securing a meaningful system of labeling in order to protect the right of consumers to avoid such foods.

Center for Media and Democracy: ___www.prwatch.org___

The nonprofit Center for Media and Democracy (CMD) is a media research group founded by environmentalist writer and political activist John Stauber. It investigates and exposes public relations spin and propaganda and by promoting media literacy and citizen journalism—media "of, by and for the people." The CMD Web site states it does not accept corporate, labor union, or government grants and favors grassroots citizen activism that promotes public health, economic justice, ecological sustainability, and human rights. Their programs include *PR Watch*, a quarterly investigative journal; books; Spin of the Day; the Weekly Spin listserv; and Congresspedia and SourceWatch.

Common Dreams: ___www.commondreams.org___

Common Dreams is a national nonprofit citizens' organization working to bring Americans together to promote progressive visions for America's future. It is committed to being on the cutting-edge of using the Internet as a political organizing tool and creating new models for Internet activism. Their "Breaking News & View for the Progressive Community" is a daily source of news, a mix of politics, issues, and breaking news with an emphasis on progressive perspectives that are increasingly hard to find with today's corporate-dominated media. The organization is funded exclusively by members and supporters with no corporate money or advertising.

CorpWatch: _www.corpwatch.org_

CorpWatch is a research group, investigating and exposing corporate violations of human rights, environmental crimes, fraud, and corruption around the world. It works to foster global justice, independent media activism, and democratic control over corporations. Founded in 1996, CorpWatch has provided journalists, activists, policy makers, students and teachers with key informational resources on issues related to corporate accountability. Today CorpWatch continues to investigate multinationals that profit out of war, fraud, environmental, and human rights abuse.

The Edmonds Institute: _www.edmonds-institute.org_

The Edmonds Institute is a nonprofit, public-interest organization committed to the health and sustainability of ecosystems and their inhabitants. It seeks to engage in projects that foster respect for and protection of the rights and health of all communities. The Institute focuses its efforts on understanding and sharing information about environmental, human rights and human health, and economic impacts of technology and intellectual property policies.

The current emphasis of its programs is on biosafety and the legally binding international regulation of modern biotechnologies, intellectual property rights and just policies for the maintenance and protection of biodiversity, including policies that foster recognition and sustenance of agricultural biodiversity, and exploration of the ethical implications of new technologies.

The Institute researches, answers inquiries from people around the world, publishes policy analyses and scientific thought pieces, sponsors public workshops, provides speakers to university and community audiences, and brings expert witnesses who share the concerns of the Institute as well as persons whose lives have been affected by technology policies to national events and to international bodies engaged in decision-making.

Fairness and Accuracy in Reporting: _www.fair.org_

Fairness and Accuracy in Reporting (FAIR), a national media-watch group, has been offering well-documented criticism of media bias and censorship since 1986. FAIR works to "invigorate the First Amendment by advocating for greater diversity in the press and by scrutinizing media practices that marginalize public interest, minority and dissenting viewpoints." As an anti-censorship organization, they expose neglected news stories and defend working journalists when they are censored. As a progressive group, FAIR believes that structural reform is ultimately needed to break up the dominant media conglomerates, establish independent public broadcasting, and promote strong nonprofit sources of information.

FAIR publishes *Extra!*, the magazine of media criticism, and produces the weekly radio program *CounterSpin* about the news behind the headlines.

Global Policy Forum: *www.globalpolicy.org*

Global Policy Forum monitors policy-making at the United Nations, promotes accountability of global decisions, educates and mobilizes for global citizen participation, and advocates on issues of international peace and justice.

Project Censored Media and Democracy in Action: *www.projectcensored.org*

Project Censored is a media research group out of Sonoma State University in California, which tracks the news published in independent journals and newsletters. Project Censored compiles an annual list of twenty-five news stories of social significance that have been overlooked, underreported, or censored by the country's major national news media.

Rachel's Environment & Health Weekly: *www.rachel.org*

Its goal is to strengthen democracy by helping people find the information they need to fight for environmental justice in their own communities. *Rachel's* believes that grassroots action is the effective lever for change in our neighborhoods and that informed citizens are the essential backbone of a strong democracy and a healthy environment.

Rachel Carson, the famous scientist and writer, published *Silent Spring* in 1962, warning that toxic industrial chemicals and pesticides would cause irreparable harm to the environment and to human health. In 1986, *Rachel's Environment & Health News* was published and named in honor of Rachel Carson. The publication provides timely information on environmental hazards. *Rachel's* puts environmental problems into a political context of money and power so people can see how the world's problems are connected. To address these concerns, it discusses issues such as the influx of money into elections, the influence of multinational corporations, and other distortions of American democracy.

Regarding U.S. Government

Capital Eye: www.capitaleye.org

Capital Eye is a money-in-politics newsletter published by the Center for Responsive Politics. Capital Eye aims to educate its readers and encourage them to examine the role of money in the U.S. political system. It includes articles on issues related to money and politics and other features designed to explore the impact of money on elections and public policy.

Center for Responsive Politics: www.opensecrets.org

The Center for Responsive Politics is a non-partisan, nonprofit research group based in Washington, D.C. that tracks money in politics and its effect on elections and public policy. The Center conducts computer-based research on campaign finance issues for the news media, academics, activists, and the public. The Center accepts no contributions from businesses or labor unions.

Environmental Commons Seed and Plant Law Preemption Tracker: http://environmentalcommons.org/gmo-tracker.html

This tracker provides up-to-date information on state legislation that impacts local sustainable farming systems and community decision-making. In response to local governments passing policies to protect family farmers and community environmental health, particularly from the impacts of GE crops, some legislators allied with the biotechnology industry and the Farm Bureau and have introduced "preemption" bills aimed at prohibiting such actions. However, many state lawmakers recognize the importance of community decision-making, local sustainable farming systems, and the impacts of GE seeds and crops.

Environmental Working Group (Farm Subsidy Database): www.ewg.org

The mission of the Environmental Working Group (EWG) is, according to its Web site, "to use the power of public information to protect public health and the environment." EWG is a nonprofit organization founded in 1993 by Ken Cook and Richard Wiles. Environmental investigations are EWG's specialty. Its team of scientists, engineers, policy experts, lawyers, and computer programmers focus on government data, legal documents, scientific studies, and its own laboratory tests to expose threats to public health and the environment and to find solutions. In addition to farm subsidy databases, the organization has also compiled databases on natural tap water contamination, mining, oil and gas leases, an auto asthma pollution level index, as well as covering other issues concerning children's health, the environment, food, water, and consumer products.

FDA Statement of Food Policy: Foods Derived from New Plant Varieties (1992): www.cfsan.fda.gov/~acrobat/ fr920529.pdf

GMO Testing

Non-GMO Project: www.nongmoproject.org

The Non-GMO Project is a nonprofit organization dedicated to enabling the public to make informed choices regarding the consumption of GE food products, achieved through a third party Non-GMO Verification Program and through outreach and education programs. The Non-GMO Project educates consumers and retailers about issues concerning GMOs in the food supply and promotes awareness about the project's non-GMO verification program, its product directory, and the meaning of its non-GMO verified "shopping cart" seal.

Non-GMO Seeds

Organic Seed Alliance: www.seedalliance.org

Organic Seed Alliance, a nonprofit public charity, supports the ethical development and stewardship of the genetic resources of agricultural seed. It accomplishes its goals through collaborative education and research programs with organic farmers and other seed professionals. You can subscribe to the quarterly e-newsletter list and receive action updates and educational workshop announcements.

Seed Savers Exchange: www.seedsavers.org

Seed Savers Exchange is a nonprofit organization that saves and shares heirloom seeds, forming a living legacy that can be passed down through generations. The organization is saving the world's diverse garden heritage for future generations by building a network of people committed to collecting, conserving, and sharing heirloom seeds and plants, while educating people about the value of genetic and cultural diversity. None of the seeds have been genetically engineered.

BOOKS

Against the Grain: Biotechnology and the Corporate Takeover of Your Food (1998) by Mark Lappé and Britt Bailey

This book cuts through biotechnology's propaganda, revealing the science and politics behind transgenic foods to show how biotech companies engineer what you eat to be compatible with their chemicals, but are not necessarily good for human health.

An Earth Saving Revolution: Volume 1 (1993) by Dr. Teruo Higa

The first book written by Dr. Teruo Higa, developer of Effective Microorganisms (EM) and Effective Microorganisms Technology. It describes Dr. Higa's discovery and the philosophy he developed through observing this product, which is now used in more than 120 countries. *An Earth Saving Revolution 1* describes how Higa first discovered EMs and how these regenerative microbial alliances can rapidly restore the health and balance of the environment.

An Earth Saving Revolution: Volume 2 (1998) by Dr. Teruo Higa

Dr. Higa's follow up to *An Earth Saving Revolution 1*, this volume offers more information about how Effective Microorganisms can be implemented in a wide variety of practical applications, such as in agriculture, the environment, and medical fields.

Dinner at the New Gene Cafe: How Genetic Engineering Is Changing What We Eat, How We Live, and the Global Politics of Food (2001) by Bill Lambrecht

Journalist Bill Lambrecht's *Dinner at the New Gene Café* follows both sides of the agricultural biotechnology debate, having interviewed agricultural officials, biotech industry executives, family farmers, and protesters to build a comprehensive understanding of the issues.

Genetic Roulette: The Documented Health Risks of Genetically Engineered Foods (2007) by Jeffrey M. Smith

Eating genetically modified food is gambling with every bite.

The biotech industry's claim that GE foods are safe is shattered in this book. Sixty-five health risks of the foods that Americans eat every day are presented in easy-to-read two-page spreads. The left page is designed for the quick scanning reader; it includes bullets, illustrations, and quotes. The right side offers fully referenced text, describing both research studies and theoretical risks. The second half of *Genetic Roulette* shows how safety assessments on GE crops are not competent to identify the health problems presented in the first half. It also exposes how industry research is rigged to avoid finding problems.

This book, prepared with input by more than thirty scientists, is for anyone wanting to understand GE technology, to learn how to protect themselves, or to share their concerns with others. As the most complete reference on the health risks of GE foods, *Genetic Roulette* is also ideal for schools and libraries. Go to www.GeneticRoulette.com for more information.

Genetically Engineered Food: A Self-Defense Guide for Consumers (2004) by Ronnie Cummins and Ben Lilliston

As food safety advocates, the authors examine scientific, political, economic, and health issues. With billions of dollars in profits at stake, the biotech food industry continues to promise that biotech will end world hunger and improve public health and the environment; however, the authors weigh those promises against the unpredictability of the new technology and the fact that much of it has not been tested for safety or labeled. Included is information on what consumers can do to reduce the threat of GE food.

Science in the Private Interest: Has the Lure of Profits Corrupted Biomedical Research? (2004) by Sheldon Krimsky

Something has changed in the culture and values of academic science; university science is now entangled with entrepreneurship, and researchers with a commercial interest are caught in an ethical quandary. *Science in the Private Interest* investigates the trends and effects of modern, commercialized academic science.

Seeds of Deception: Exposing Industry and Government Lies About the Safety of the Genetically Engineered Foods You're Eating (2003) by Jeffrey M. Smith

Jeffrey M. Smith's international bestseller and exposé reveals "what the biotech industry doesn't want you to know": how industry manipulation and political collusion, not sound science, have allowed dangerous genetically engineered food into the American daily diet virtually undetected. Examples of how company research is rigged, alarming evidence of health dangers is covered up, and intense political pressure applied are numerous. Smith offers cases where GE food produced unexpected scientific results—from increased starch content in potatoes to pigs without genitals. He describes a clear picture of how GE foods made their way into the food supply and how conflicts of interest, questionable science, and industry influence affected the approval process of GE food in America.

The 2007 Non-GMO Sourcebook by Writing Solutions, Inc.

This book features more than six hundred non-GMO suppliers and service providers, including seed companies, growers, grain suppliers, exporters, processors, ingredient manufacturers, food manufacturers, GMO testing labs, GMO test-kit manufacturers, identity preservation, consultants, organic certifiers, and more. You can order *The 2007 Non-GMO Sourcebook* from www.non-gmoreport.com.

The Biotech Century: Harnessing the Gene and Remaking the World (1998) by Jeremy Rifkin

Rifkin addresses recombinant DNA techniques, computer gene mapping, and the globalization of commerce that affects our lives. Though he does not dispute the possible benefits of biotechnology, Rifkin, president of the Foundation on Economic Trends and author of many other books, says we must consider its possible adverse effects. He asserts that biotechnology has the ability to deplete the planet's gene pool and irreparably damage ecological balance. Just as the Industrial Revolution caused unexpected problems, such as depletion of natural resources, overpopulation, economic injustice, and pollution, the Biotech Revolution will also cause problems we cannot yet imagine.

The Food Revolution: How Your Diet Can Help Save Your Life and Our World (2001) by John Robbins

Author of *Diet for a New America*, John Robbins believes that plant-based nutrition and particularly vegan diets (free of meat, milk, and eggs) lead to long life and good health. In *The Food Revolution*, Robbins devotes a section to genetically engineered food as part of a broad picture of agricultural factory farming today.

Trust Us We're Experts: How Industry Manipulates Science and Gambles with Your Future (2001) by Sheldon Rampton and John Stauber

Investigative journalists Sheldon Rampton's and John Stauber's *Trust Us* is an exposé of the public relations industry and the scientists who support their corporate agendas, sometimes at the risk of public health. The authors reveal two kinds of "experts" who can fool the public: the public relations talking heads behind the scenes and the "independent" scientific experts who have been carefully selected and paid well to promote the views of corporations.

What's In Your Milk?: An Exposé of Industry and Government Cover-Up on the Dangers of the Genetically Engineered (rBGH) Milk You're Drinking (2007) by Samuel S. Epstein, M.D.

Epstein's exposé shows the dangers, especially to children, of non-organic milk contaminated by a GE growth hormone (rBGH) without any warning of its difference from natural milk, and of its cancer risks. Supported by the FDA, Monsanto insists that rBGH milk is indistinguishable from natural milk and that it is safe.

Epstein reveals the truth about rBGH: that it makes cows sick, and Monsanto has been forced to admit to about twenty toxic effects on its Posilac label; that rBGH milk is contaminated by pus due to the mastitis commonly induced by rBGH and antibiotics used to treat the mastitis; that it is chemically and nutritionally different than natural milk; and that traces of rBGH are absorbed through the gut, charged with high levels of a natural growth factor (IGF-1), which has been incriminated as a cause of breast, colon, and prostate cancers. Overall, it shows that rBGH enriches Monsanto, while posing dangers, without any benefits, to consumers, especially in view of the current national surplus of milk.

Epstein is professor emeritus of environmental and occupational medicine at the University of Illinois School of Public Health and chair of the Cancer Prevention Coalition. He has published some 260 peer-reviewed articles and authored or co-authored eleven books, including: the prize-winning 1978 *The Politics of*

Cancer; the 1998 *Breast Cancer Prevention Program*; the 1998 *The Politics of Cancer, Revisited*; the 2001 *GOT (Genetically Engineered) MILK! The Monsanto rBGH/BST Milk Wars Handbook*; the 2001 *Unreasonable Risk*, and others.

World's Wasted Wealth 2: Save Our Wealth, Save Our Environment (1994) by Dr. J.W. Smith

"We all want a peaceful and prosperous world, yet nations continually battle over the world's wealth and keep the world impoverished," says Smith. This book is an analysis of the enormous waste of labor, resources, and capital within the American economy.

FILM DOCUMENTARIES

Islands at Risk: Genetic Engineering in Hawaii (2006), Na Maka o ka 'Aina: www.namaka.com/catalog/environment/ genetic.html

Hawaii has been called the GE-testing capitol of the world with more than two thousand field tests of experimental GE crops in more than six thousand (undisclosed) locations.

This video/DVD was produced for Earthjustice, a non-profit public interest law firm, by Na Maka o ka 'Aina ("The Eyes of the Land"), an independent video production team that focuses on the land and the people of Hawaii and the Pacific. Earthjustice has won lawsuits in federal and state courts, challenging the introduction of these experimental crop tests on the islands without first assessing the environmental and human health impacts. The 30-minute film can be viewed in its entirety online at: www.warthjustice.org/news/multimedia/video1/ page.jsp?itemID=29841806 or visit www.namaka.com/catalog/environment/ genetic.html to purchase the video DVD.

The Future of Food (2004) by Deborah Garcia, Lily Films: www.thefutureoffood.com

This documentary explores the disturbing truth behind the unlabeled, patented, GE foods that have become part of the American diet for the past decade. Filmed on location in the United States, Canada, and Mexico, *The Future of Food* examines the market and political forces that have changed what we eat, while multinational corporations attempt to control the world's food system. The film also explores alternatives to large-scale industrial agriculture.

Notes

Introduction: Americans Kept in the Dark

1. Pollan, Michael. "Playing God in the Garden." Organic Consumers Association, originally released in the *New York Times* (October 25, 1998). www.organicconsumers.org/ge/playinggd.htm

2. *Statement of Food Policy: Foods Derived from New Plant Varieties.* FDA *Federal Register*, Vol. 57, No. 104, p. 22991 (May 29, 1992). http://www.cfsan.fda.gov/~acrobat/fr920529.pdf

3. *Review of FDA/Industry Consultations Regarding New Plant Varieties and Selectable Markers Used to Develop Them. Appendix 2: Purpose of the Consultations.* FDA Guidance for Industry: Use of Antibiotic Resistance Marker Genes in Transgenic Plants (September 4, 1998). http://www.cfsan.fda.gov/~dms/opa-armg.html

4. *Statement of Food Policy: Foods Derived from New Plant Varieties.* FDA *Federal Register*, Vol. 57, No. 104, p. 22991 (May 29, 1992). http://www.cfsan.fda.gov/~acrobat/fr920529.pdf

5. Pollan, Michael. "Playing God in the Garden." Organic Consumers Association, originally released in the *New York Times* (October 25, 1998). www.organicconsumers.org/ge/playinggd.htm

6. Smith, Jeffrey M. "Most Offspring Died When Mother Rats Ate Genetically Engineered Soy." *Spilling the Beans* Newsletter (October 2005). http://www.seedsofdeception.com/utility/showArticle/?objectID=297

7. Ibid.

8. *The Future of Food*, VHS/DVD, written, directed and produced by Deborah Garcia (2004); Lily Films.

9. *Comments on Proposed Draft Guidelines for the Labeling of Food and Food Ingredients Obtained Through Certain Techniques of Genetic Modification/Genetic Engineering: Labeling Provisions (At Step 3 of the Procedure).* Consumers International (March 2005). http://www.consumersinternational.org/shared_asp_files/uploadedfiles/A15E8C64-0BE3-480E-BD7B-1331A22B90D5_CIstatement.doc

10. Weiss, Rick. "U.S. Uneasy about Biotech Food, Americans Lack Knowledge, Faith in FDA's Accuracy, Poll Finds." *Washington Post*, p. A16 (December

7, 2006). http://www.washingtonpost.com/wp-dyn/content/article/2006/12/06/AR2006120601349.html

11. Davoudi, Salamander. "Monsanto: Giant of the $6.15bn GM Market." *Financial Times* (November 16, 2006). http://www.organicconsumers.org/2006/article_3393.cfm

12. Lambrecht, Bill & Shesgreen, Dierdre. "Monsanto Continues to Block Federal Legislation on Labeling & Safety Testing of GE Foods & Crops." Organic Consumers Association (September 12, 2005). http://www.organicconsumers.org/monsanto/safety091305.cfm

13. "Why Biotech Labeling Can Confuse Consumers." Council for Biotechnology Information (2004). http://www.whybiotech.com/index.asp?id=1811

Chapter 1: The Biotech Façade

1. *The Future of Food*, VHS/DVD, written, directed and produced by Deborah Garcia (2004); Lily Films.

2. Robbins, John. *The Food Revolution: How Your Diet Can Help Save Your Life and the World*, p. 331. Berkeley, CA: Conari Press, 2001.

3. "Genetically Engineered Food." Center for Food Safety (2005). http://www.centerforfoodsafety.org/geneticall7.cfm

4. Suurkula, Jaan. "Junk DNA: Over 95 Percent of DNA has Largely Unknown Function." Physicians and Scientists for Responsible Application of Science and Technology (PSRAST) (2003). http://www.psrast.org/junkdna.htm

5. Cummins, Ronnie & Lilliston, Ben. *Genetically Engineered Food*, p. 18. New York, NY: Marlowe & Company, 2004.

6. Suzuki, David. "Biotechnology: A Geneticist's Perspective." http://www.davidsuzuki.org/files/general/dtsbiotech.pdf. Permission to quote was granted to the author from Dr. Suzuki.

7. Ibid.

8. Smith, Jeffrey M. "Scrambling and Gambling with the Genome." *Spilling the Beans* Newsletter (July 2005). http://www.seedsofdeception.com/Public/Newsletter/July05ScramblingtheGenome/index.cfm

9. Smith, Jeffrey M. *Genetic Roulette: The Documented Health Risks of Genetically Engineered Foods*, pp. 3-4. White River Junction, Vermont: Chelsea Green Publishing, 2007. Author received permission from Jeffrey M. Smith to reprint analogy in its entirety.

10. Drucker, Steven. "Alliance for Bio-Integrity Lawsuit Overview." Alliance for Bio-Integrity (2005). http://www.biointegrity.org/Overview.html

11. U.S. Supreme Court, *Diamond v. Chakrabarty, 447 U.S. 303* (1980). FindLaw for Legal Professionals. http://caselaw.lp.findlaw. com/scripts/getcase.pl?court=us&vol=447&invol=303

12. Rifkin, Jeremy. *The Biotech Century: Harnessing the Gene and Remaking the World*, p. 43. New York, NY: Tarcher/Putnam, 1998.

13. Ibid., 48.

14. Ibid., 44.

15. "Genetically Engineered Food." Center for Food Safety (2005). http://www.centerforfoodsafety.org/geneticall7.cfm

16. *The Future of Food*, VHS/DVD, written, directed and produced by Deborah Garcia (2004); Lily Films.

17. Monsanto Company (2005). www.monsanto.com

18. Agent Orange Lawsuit (2005). http://www.agent-orange-lawsuit.com/

19. "EPA Investigates Monsanto." *Rachel's Environment & Health News #400* (July 27, 1994). http://www.rachel.org/bulletin/pdf/Rachels_Environment_Health_News_727.pdf

20. Cox, Carolyn. "Glyphosate, Part 2: Human Exposure and Ecological Effects." *Journal of Pesticide Reform* (v.108, n.3 Fall 98 rev.Oct 00). Mindfully.org   http://www.mindfully.org/Pesticide/Roundup-Glyphosate-Factsheet-Cox2.htm and "Some Health Consequences of Roundup Poisoning" originally printed in *The Ecologist* Vol. 28 No. 5 (June 27, 1999). http://ecolu-info.unige.ch/archives/envcee99/0183.html

21. Miller, Karl, M.D. "Pesticide Exposure and Non-Hodgkin's Lymphoma." American Academy of Family Physicians (August 1999). http://www.aafp.org/afp/990800ap/tips/17.html

22. Richard, Sophie, Moslemi, Safa, Sipahutar, Herbert, Benachour, Nora, & Seralini, Gilles-Eric. "Differential Effects of Glyphosate and Roundup on Human Placental Cells and Aromatase." *Environmental Health Perspectives* (June 2005). http://ehp.niehs.nih.gov/docs/2005/7728/abstract.html

23. Relyea, Rick. "The Lethal Impact of Roundup on Aquatic and Terrestrial Amphibians." *Ecological Society of America, Ecological Applications*, Vol. 15, Issue 4, pp. 1118-1124 (August 2005). http://www.esajournals.org/esaonline/?request=get-abstract&issn=1051-0761&volume=015&issue=04&page=1118

24. Monsanto Company (2005). www.monsanto.com

25. Green, Che. "The Unwholesome Collusion of the USDA, Monsanto, and the U.S. Dairy Industry." *Lip Magazine* (May 25, 2002). http://www.lipmagazine.org/articles/featgreen_172.shtml

26. "Dairy Program Subsidies in the United States." Environmental Working Group Farm Subsidy Database (2005). http://www.ewg.org/farm/progdetail.php?fips=00000&progcode=dairy

27. Teather, David. "Monsanto Found Guilty of Polluting." Ethical Investing.com, originally released in *The Guardian* (February 25, 2002). http://www.ethicalinvesting.com/monsanto/news/10074.htm

28. Ibid.

29. "Environmental Justice Case Study: The People of Anniston, Alabama vs. Monsanto." University of Michigan School of Natural Resources and Environment (2002). http://www.umich.edu/~snre492/Jones/anniston.htm

30. Krishnakumar, Asha. "A Multinational Exposed." *Frontline* (Vol. 22, Issue 05, February 26–March 11, 2005). http://www.frontlineonnet.com/fl2205/stories/20050311003312500.htm

31. Richardson, Len. "Monsanto's Salad Taste; Mean Bite Feeds Growth." *California Farmer* (March 2005), p. 7.

32. Flint, James. "Agricultural Industry Giants Moving Towards Genetic Monopolism." *Telepolis* (June 28, 1998). http://www.heise.de/tp/r4/artikel/2/2385/1.html

33. Culp, Craig. "Monsanto's Assault on U.S. Farmers Detailed in New Report." Center for Food Safety (2005). http://www.percyschmeiser.com/MonsantovsFarmers.htm; a PDF of the entire report *Monsanto vs. U.S. Farmers* is available at http://www.percyschmeiser.com/MonsantovsFarmerReport1.13.05.pdf

34. Richardson, Len. "Monsanto's Salad Taste; Mean Bite Feeds Growth." *California Farmer* (March 2005), p. 7.

35. Gillam, Carey. "Crop King Monsanto Seeks Pig-Breeding Patent Clout." Common Dreams, originally released by Reuters (August 10, 2005). http://www.commondreams.org/headlines05/0810-04.htm

36. Syngenta Company (2005). http://www.syngenta.com/en/index.aspx

37. Shiva, Vandana. "The Golden Rice Hoax: When Public Relations Replaces Science." San Francisco State University Online (October 26, 2000). http://online.sfsu.edu/~rone/GEessays/goldenricehoax.html

38. "Syngenta the Biotech Giant Wants to Own Our Food." Swissaid Media Release (August 11, 2005). Organic Consumers Association. http://www.organicconsumers.org/ge/syngenta081605.cfm

39. "Syngenta Breaks Promise on Development of Terminator Genetically Modified Plants; Seed Giant Applies to Field Test." GM Food News (July 25, 2001). http://www.gmfoodnews.com/gm250701.txt

40. "Swiss Biotech Giant Syngenta Sold Hundreds of Tons of Non-Approved GE Corn to U.S." Organic Consumers Association, originally released by Reuters (March 22, 2005). http://www.organicconsumers.org/ge/syngenta032305.cfm

41. "GMO Corn Blockade—German Consumer Protection Minister: 'Unbelievable Sloppiness!'" *Der Spiegel* (Speigel Online) (April 18, 2005). http://service.spiegel.de/cache/international/spiegel/0,1518,352006,00.html

42. "Syngenta the Biotech Giant Wants to Own Our Food." Swissaid Media Release (August 11, 2005). Organic Consumers Association. http://www.organicconsumers.org/ge/syngenta081605.cfm

43. Ibid.

44. Bayer CropScience (2005). http://www.bayercropscience.com

45. Pollack, Andrew. "Aventis & EPA Knew Banned Starlink Corn Was Getting Into Food Supply." Organic Consumers Association, originally released in the *New York Times* (September 4, 2001). http://www.organicconsumers.org/gefood/starlink090501.cfm

46. Bayer CropScience (2005). http://www.bayercropscience.com

47. "Top Scientific Journal Admits Transgenic Crop Contamination is Inevitable." Organic Consumers Association, originally released in *Nature* (January 10, 2007). http://www.organicconsumers.org/articles/article_3806.cfm

48. "Bayer CropScience: Sales of new products should rise to € 2 billion." Bayer CropScience (September 5, 2005). http://www.bayercropscience.com/bayer/cropscience/cscms.nsf/id/351984D1350F00FAC12570C70039AC77

49. "Bayer Reaches Settlement over Drug Disclosure." *Houston Business Journal* (January 23, 2007). http://houston.bizjournals.com/houston/stories/2007/01/22/daily29.html

50. "DuPont: Overview." Corporate Watch, Oxford, United Kingdom (November 2002). http://www.corporatewatch.org/?lid=170

51. "DuPont's Path to Biotechnology." *Delaware Online News Journal* (August 14, 2005). http://www.delawareonline.com/apps/pbcs.dll/article?AID=/20050814/NEWS01/508140335/1006

52. DuPont Biotechnology (2005). http://www2.dupont.com/Biotechnology/en_US/

53. Barnett, Antony. "Eyeless Children Championed by The Observer Win $7m Test Case." GM Food News, originally released in *The Observer* (December 21, 2003). http://www.gmfoodnews.com/ob211203.txt

54. Ibid.

55. Ibid.

56. Ward Jr., Ken. "DuPont Proposed, Dropped '81 Study of C8, Birth Defects." *Teflon Consumer Alert*, originally released in *The Charleston Gazette* (July 10, 2005). http://www.teflonconsumeralert.org/Teflon_Consumer_Alert_WORD_files/DuPont_Charleston_Gazette_July_10.doc

57. Hawthorne, Michael. "U.S. Officials Accuse DuPont of Concealing Teflon Ingredient's Health Risk." Environmental News Network, originally released in the *Chicago Tribune* (January 18, 2005). http://www.enn.com/today.html?id=6949

58. "DuPont's Path to Biotechnology." *Delaware Online News Journal* (August 14, 2005). http://www.delawareonline.com/apps/pbcs.dll/article?AID=/20050814/NEWS01/508140335/1006

59. Freese, Bill. "Genetically Modified Crops Still Not Performing: New Report Dispels Decade of Hype from Biotech Industry." Center for Food Safety (January 9, 2007). http://www.centerforfoodsafety.org/WhoBenefits_PR_1_9_07.cfm

60. Leahy, Stephen. "GE Crops Slow to Gain Global Acceptance." Common Dreams (January 10, 2007). www.commondreams.org/headlines07/0110-06.htm

61. *Seeds of Doubt: North American Farmers' Experiences of GM Crops.* The Soil Association (2002), p. 4. PDF available from Greenpeace.org. http://www.greenpeace.org/raw/content/international/press/reports/seeds-of-doubt-north-american.pdf

62. Leahy, Stephen. "GE Crops Slow to Gain Global Acceptance." Common Dreams (January 10, 2007). www.commondreams.org/headlines07/0110-06.htm

63. "Ten Reasons Why GE Crops Won't Feed the World." Corner House (1998). http://www.thecornerhouse.org.uk/item.shtml?x=52221 #index-10-00-00-00

64. "Briefing: Genetically Modified Food." Friends of the Earth (June 2001). http://www.foe.co.uk/resource/briefings/gm_food.html#Footref36

65. Smith, J.W. *The World's Wasted Wealth II*, pp. 63-64. Cambria, California: The Institute for Economic Democracy, 1994.

66. Kirby, Alex. "Mirage of GM's Golden Promise." Biotech-Info.net, originally released by BBC News (February 2004). http://www.biotech-info.net/mirage_of_promise.html

67. Robbins, John. *The Food Revolution: How Your Diet Can Help Save Your Life and the World*, pp. 317-318. Berkeley, CA: Conari Press, 2001.

68. Bereano, Philip. "Engineered-Food Claims are Hard to Swallow." Common Dreams, originally released by the *Seattle Times* (November 19, 2002). http://www.commondreams.org/views02/1119-03.htm

69. Patel, Rajeev, Torres, Robert, & Rosset, Peter. "Genetic Engineering in Agriculture and Corporate Engineering in Public Debate: Risk, Public Relations, and Public Debate over Genetically Modified Crops." *International Journal of Occupational and Environmental Health* (2005). http://www.ijoeh.com/pfds/IJOEH_1104_Patel.pdf

70. Nord, Mark, Andrews, Margaret, & Carlson, Stephen. *Household Food Security in the United States, 2005.* Economic Research Service Report (October 2005). http://www.ers.usda.gov/Publications/err11/

71. Fernandez-Cornejo, Jorge, & McBride, William. *The Adoption of Bioengineered Crops.* Economic Research Service Report (May 2002), p. 30. http://www.ers.usda.gov/publications/aer810/

72. Griffiths, Mark. "The Emperor's Transgenic Clothes: Are GMO Lemmings in the U.S. Leading All of Us Over the Biotechnology Cliff?" Natural Law Party Wessex (May 1999). http://www.btinternet.com/~nlpwessex/Documents/gmlemmings.htm

73. Ibid.

74. Lambert, Charles. "Biotech Products Rigorously Regulated." U.S. Department of State speech to Senate Agriculture Committee (June 15, 2005). http://usinfo.state.gov/ei/Archive/2005/Jun/16-474089.html

75. "GM Safety Tests Flawed—New Research." Friends of the Earth (November 16, 2004). http://www.foe.co.uk/resource/press_releases/gm_safety_tests_flawed_new_24112004.html

76. Pollack, Andrew. "U.S. Agency Violated Law in Seed Case, Judge Rules." The Campaign, originally released in the *New York Times* (February 14, 2007). http://www.thecampaign.org/forums/showthread.php?t=505

77. Maryanski, James. "Statement on Biotechnology Issues." Speech before the Senate Committee on Agriculture, Nutrition and Forestry. (October 7, 1999). http://www.hhs.gov/asl/testify/t991007a.html

78. Ibid.

79. Ibid.

80. Pollan, Michael. "Playing God in the Garden." Organic Consumers Association, originally released in the *New York Times* Sunday Magazine (October 25, 1998). www.organicconsumers.org/ge/playinggd.htm

81. "FDA Names Food Safety Czar." HealthCentral.com, originally released by Reuters (May 2, 2007). http://www.healthcentral.com/diet-exercise/news-38122-66.html

82. Ibid.

83. "GM Safety Tests Flawed—New Research." Friends of the Earth (November 16, 2004). http://www.foe.co.uk/resource/press_releases/gm_safety_tests_flawed_new_24112004.html

84. Ibid.

85. "Genetically Altering the World's Food." *Rachel's Democracy & Health News* #639 (February 25, 1999). http://www.rachel.org/bulletin/bulletin.cfm?Issue_ID=1282

86. Robbins, John. *The Food Revolution: How Your Diet Can Help Save Your Life and the World*, p. 324. Berkeley, CA: Conari Press, 2001.

87. Woolf, Marie. "Emergency Planning to Cope with GM Bio-Disasters." Mothers for Natural Law, originally released in *The Independent* (April 16, 1999). http://www.safe-food.org/-news/1999-04-16.html

88. "Farmers Told GM Crops 'Too Dangerous to Insure.'" Mindfully.org, originally released in *The Herald (UK)* (March 10, 2002). http://www.mindfully.org/GE/GE4/Too-Dangerous-To-Insure10mar02.htm

Chapter 2: Science Under the Influence

1. Pribyl, Dr. Louis, Memorandum to James Maryanski, the FDA's biotech coordinator regarding Federal Register draft document, *Statement of Policy: Foods from Genetically Modified Plants*. Alliance for Bio-Integrity (February 27, 1992). http://www.biointegrity.org/FDAdocs/04/view1.html

2. Rampton, Sheldon & Stauber, John. *Trust Us, We're Experts: How Industry Manipulates Science and Gambles with Your Future*, p. 189. New York, NY: Tarcher/Putnam, 2001.

3. "Scientific Integrity in Policy Making." Union of Concerned Scientists (2005). http://www.ucsusa.org/scientific_integrity/

4. Lightfoot, Liz. "Scientists Asked to Fix Results for Backer." GM Watch, originally released in the *London Telegraph* (February 14, 2000). http://www.gmwatch.org/archive2.asp?arcid=5354

5. Library of Congress, Federal Technology Transfer Act (1986). http://thomas.loc.gov/cgi-bin/bdquery/z?d099:HR03773:@@@L&summ2=m&%7CTOM:/bss/d099query.html

6. Rifkin, Jeremy. *The Biotech Century: Harnessing the Gene and Remaking the World*, p. 56. New York, NY: Tarcher/Putnam, 1998.

7. Rampton, Sheldon, & Stauber, John. *Research Funding, Conflicts of Interest, and the Meta-methodology of Public Relations.* Public Health Report (July-August 2002). www.publichealthreports.org/userfiles/117_4/117331.pdf

8. Klotz-Ingram, Cassandra & Day-Rubenstein, Kelly. "The Changing Agricultural Research Environment: What Does it Mean for Public-Private Innovation? *USDA AgBioForum*, Vol. 2, No. 1, Article 5 (1999). http://www.agbioforum.org/v2n1/v2n1a05-klotz.htm

9. Hord, Bill. "Regent Calls Pact Raw Deal for Farmers." Say No To GMOs, originally released in the *Knight-Ridder Tribune* (March 25, 2005). http://www.saynotogmos.org/ud2005/umar05c.html#dicamba

10. Frenay, Robert. "Biotech—Impure Research." *Pulse* (April 9, 2006). http://www.pulsethebook.com/index.php/index.php?tag=biotech

11. Ibid.

12. Krimsky, Sheldon & Rothenberg, L.S. "Conflict of Interest Policies in Science and Medical Journals: Editorial Practices and Author Disclosures." *Science and Engineering Ethics* (2001), 7, 205-218. http://www.tufts.edu/~skrimsky/PDF/conflict.PDF

13. Blumenthal, D., Campbell, E.G., Anderson, M.S., Causino, N., & Louis, K.S. "Withholding Research Results in Academic Life Science. Evidence from a National Survey of Faculty." *Journal of the American Medical Association* (April 16, 1997). http://jama.ama-assn.org/cgi/content/abstract/277/15/1224

14. Suzuki, David. "Biotechnology: A Geneticist's Personal Perspective." http://www.davidsuzuki.org/files/general/dtsbiotech.pdf

15. Ross, John. "The Sad Saga of Ignacio Chapela." *The Anderson Valley Advertiser* (February 18, 2004). www.theava.com/04/0218-chapela.html

16. Locke, Michelle. "Biologist Protests his Lack of Tenure." Mindfully.org, originally released by the Associated Press (June 27, 2003). http://www.mindfully.org/GE/2003/Ignacio-Chapela-Tenure27jun03.htm

17. Ross, John. "The Sad Saga of Ignacio Chapela." *The Anderson Valley Advertiser* (February 18, 2004). www.theava.com/04/0218-chapela.html

18. Rampton, Sheldon & Stauber, John. *Trust Us, We're Experts: How Industry Manipulates Science and Gambles with Your Future*, pp. 153-154. New York, NY: Tarcher/Putnam, 2001.

19. Hammond, B., Vicini, J.L., Hartnell, G.F., Naylor, M.W., Knight, C.D., Robinson, E.H., Fuchs, R.L., & Padgette, S.R. "The Feeding Value of Soybeans Fed to Rats, Chickens, Catfish and Dairy Cattle is Not Altered by Genetic Incorporation of Glyphosate Tolerance." *Journal of Nutrition* (March 1996), 126(3),

717-27. http://www.ncbi.nlm.nih.gov/sites/entrez?cmd=Retrieve&db= PubMed&list_uids=8598557&dopt=Abstract

20. Rampton, Sheldon & Stauber, John. *Trust Us, We're Experts: How Industry Manipulates Science and Gambles with Your Future*, pp. 153-154. New York, NY: Tarcher/Putnam, 2001.

21. Ibid.

22. Pusztai, Arpad & Ewen, W.B. "Effect of Diets Containing Genetically Modified Potatoes Expressing Galanthus nivalis Lectin on Rat Small Intestine." Biotech-info.net, originally released in *The Lancet* (October 13, 1999), 354, 1353-1354. http://www.biotech-info.net/galanthus.html

23. Rampton, Sheldon & Stauber, John. *Trust Us, We're Experts: How Industry Manipulates Science and Gambles with Your Future*, p. 158. New York, NY: Tarcher/Putnam, 2001.

24. Pusztai, Arpad & Ewen, W.B. "Effect of Diets Containing Genetically Modified Potatoes Expressing Galanthus nivalis Lectin on Rat Small Intestine." Biotech-info.net, originally released in *The Lancet* (October 13, 1999), 354, 1353-1354. http://www.biotech-info.net/galanthus.html

25. Brown, Colin. "Suppressed Report Shows Cancer Link to GM Potatoes." *The Independent* (February 17, 2007). http://news.independent.co.uk/health/article2278044.ece

26. Ibid.

27. Krimsky, S., Rothenberg, L.S., Stott, P., & Kyle, G. "Scientific Journals and Their Authors' Financial Interests: A Pilot Study." *Psychotherapy and Psychosomatics.* (July-October 1998), 67(4-5), 194-201. http://www.ncbi.nlm.nih.gov/sites/entrez?cmd=Retrieve&db=PubMed&list_uids=9693346&dopt=Abstract

28. Krimsky, Sheldon & Rothenberg, L.S. "Conflict of Interest Policies in Science and Medical Journals: Editorial practices and Author Disclosures." *Science and Engineering Ethics* (April 26, 2001) 7, 205-218. http://www.tufts.edu/~skrimsky/PDF/conflict.PDF

29. "Journal Editors Urged to Disclose Conflicts of Interest." Center for Science in the Public Interest (August 21, 2003). http://cspinet.org/new/200308211.html

30. Nading, Tanya. "Conflicts of Interest in Biomedical Publishing: A Discussion with Sheldon Krimsky." Science Editor (July-August 2005), Vol. 28, No. 4, pp. 117-119. http://www.councilscienceeditors.org/members/secured Documents/v28n4p117-119.pdf

31. "Court Orders Monsanto to Make Scandal Report Public." Greenpeace International (June 10, 2005). http://www.greenpeace.org/international/press/releases/0610-Monsanto_court_case_Germany

32. *13-Week Dietary Subchronic Comparison Study with MON 863 Corn in Rats Preceded by a 1-Week Baseline Food Consumption Determination with PMI Certified Rodent Diet #5002.* Monsanto's Full Rat Study Report MSL 18175 (MON863). (December 17, 2002). http://www.monsanto. com/monsanto/content/sci_tech/prod_safety/fullratstudy.pdf

33. "Court Orders Monsanto to Make Scandal Report Public." Greenpeace International (June 10, 2005). http://www.greenpeace.org/international/press/releases/0610-Monsanto_court_case_Germany

34. Smith, Jeffrey M. Seeds of Deception (2005). http://www.seedsofdeception.com

35. Ibid.

36. Drucker, Steven M. "Landmark Lawsuit Challenges FDA Policy on Genetically Engineered Food." Alliance for Bio-Integrity (2001). http://www.biointegrity.org/Lawsuit.html.

37. Ibid.

38. Pribyl, Dr. Louis, Memorandum to James Maryanski, the FDA's biotech coordinator regarding Federal Register draft document, *Statement of Policy: Foods from Genetically Modified Plants.* Alliance for Bio-Integrity (February 27, 1992). http://www.biointegrity.org/FDAdocs/04/view1.html

39. Kahl, Linda, Memorandum to James Maryanski, the FDA's biotech coordinator regarding Federal Register draft document, *Statement of Policy: Foods from Genetically Modified Plants.* Alliance for Bio-Integrity (January 8, 1992). http://www.biointegrity.org/FDAdocs/01/view1.html

40. Regal, Ph.D., Philip J. "Declaration Regarding Alliance for Bio-Integrity, et. al Plaintiffs v. Donna Shalala, et. al Defendants, Civil Action No. 98-1300 (CKK)." Alliance for BioIntegrity (May 28, 1999). http://www.biointegrity.org/regaldeclaration.html

41. Drucker, Steven M. "Landmark Lawsuit Challenges FDA Policy on Genetically Engineered Food." Alliance for Bio-Integrity (2001). http://www.biointegrity.org/Lawsuit.html.

42. *Statement of Food Policy: Foods Derived from New Plant Varieties.* FDA *Federal Register*, Vol. 57, No. 104, p. 22991 (May 29, 1992). http://www.cfsan.fda.gov/~acrobat/fr920529.pdf

43. Drucker, Steven M. "Landmark Lawsuit Challenges FDA Policy on Genetically Engineered Food." Alliance for Bio-Integrity (2001). http://www.biointegrity.org/Lawsuit.html.

44. Drucker, Steven M. *How a U.S. District Court Revealed the Unsoundness of the FDA's Policy on Genetically Engineered Foods.* Alliance for Bio-Integrity Lawsuit Report, Alliance for Bio-Integrity (October 1, 2003). http://www. biointegrity.org/report-on-lawsuit.htm

45. Montague, Peter. "The Wingspread Statement on the Precautionary Principle." Mindfully.org., originally released in *Rachel's Environment & Health Weekly #586* (February 19, 1998). http://www.mindfully.org/Precaution/ Precautionary-Principle-Rachels.htm

46. Personal correspondence via e-mail with Worku Damena Yifru, Programme Officer, Policy and Legal Biosafety Division, Secretariat, Convention on Biological Diversity, United Nations Environment Programme, Canada. (January 26, 2007).

47. "Health Effects of GM Foods Need Further Study, WHO Says." Food Navigator—USA (June 24, 2005). http://www.foodnavigatorusa.com/news/ printNewsBis.asp?id=60866

48. "Politics, Not Science, Informed Policy that Leaves Engineered Foods Untested and Unlabeled." Center for Food Safety (June 7, 2006). http:// www.centerforfoodsafety.org/Ge_Foods_FDA_Complaint6_7_2006.cfm

49. *Department of Health and Human Services Docket No. 2000P-1211/CP1* (August 25, 2006). Response to Citizens Petition lodged by Center for Food Safety. Document: FDA Petition Answer 8-25-06.pdf was e-mailed to author from legal director Joseph Mendelson, Center for Food Safety.

50. Dairy Program Subsidies in the United States. Environmental Working Group, Farm Subsidy Database (2005). http://www.ewg.org/farm/ progdetail.php?fips=00000&progcode=dairy

51. Cohen, Robert. "Report on FDA Lawsuit on rBGH." *Not Milk* Newsletter (January 3, 1999). http:///www.notmilk.com/deb/010399.html. And Cohen, Robert. *MILK: The Deadly Poison*, p.93. Englewood Cliffs, NJ: Argus Publishing Inc, 1998.

52. "Leading Advocates Against Genetically Modified rBGH Milk File Citizens' Petition with FDA." The Campaign, originally released by PRNewswire-USNewswire (February 21, 2007). http://www.thecampaign.org/forums/ showthread.php?t=519

53. Cohen, Mitchell. "Got Pus? Bovine Growth Hormone, Genetic Engineering and the New World Order." Mindfully.org (August 13, 2001). http://www.mindfully.org/GE/GE3/rBGH-Got-Pus.htm

54. *U.S. Census Bureau, Statistical Abstract of the United States: 2007, Section 3, Health and Nutrition.* http://www.census.gov/prod/2006pubs/07statab/health.pdf

55. Pulaski, Alex. "Tillamook Dairies Uphold Hormone Ban; The Creamery Association Rejects a Change in Bylaws Supported by Posilac Maker Monsanto." Say No to GMOs, originally released in *The Oregonian* (March 1, 2005). http://www.saynotogmos.org/ud2005/umar05.html

56. McCall, William. "Dairy Co-op Rejects Monsanto Proposal to Drop Hormone Ban." GM Watch, originally released by The Associated Press (March 1, 2005). http://www.gmwatch.org/archive2.asp?arcid=4930

57. Gillam, Carey. "Monsanto Cites Milk Tests, Says Consumers Being Misled." Organic Consumers Association, originally released by Reuters (January 25, 2007). http://www.organicconsumers.org/articles/article_3911.cfm

58. "Americans Clueless about Gene-Altered Foods." Mindfully.org, originally released by the Associated Press (March 23, 2005). http://www.mindfully.org/GE/2005/Americans-Clueless-GMOs23mar05.htm

59. Ho, Mae-Wan. "Report on Horizontal Gene Transfer." Institute for Science in Society (March 22, 1999). http://www.i-sis.org.uk/ireaff99.php. Permission to quote was granted to the author by Sam Burcher on behalf of Dr. Ho.

60. Ibid.

61. Ibid.

62. *The Future of Food*, VHS/DVD, written, directed and produced by Deborah Garcia (2004); Lily Films.

63. *State of Programs—Foods and Human Drugs.* FDA FY 1998 Accomplishments (2000). http://www.fda.gov/oc/oms/ofm/budget/2000/fooddrugstat.htm

64. Robbins, John. *The Food Revolution: How Your Diet Can Help Save Your Life and the World*, p. 333. Berkeley, CA: Conari Press, 2001.

65. Ibid.

66. Pusztai, Arpad. "Genetically Modified Foods: Are They a Risk to Human/Animal Health?" Action Bio-Science (2001). http://www.actionbioscience.org/biotech/pusztai.html

67. "Food Related Diseases." Centers for Disease Control (2003). http://www.cdc.gov/ncidod/diseases/food/index.htm

68 "Foodborne Illness, Frequently Asked Questions." Centers for Disease Control (January 10, 2005). http://www.cdc.gov/ncidod/dbmd/diseaseinfo/files/foodborne_illness_FAQ.pdf

69. Ho, Mae-Wan. "U.S. Foodborne Illnesses Up Two to Ten Fold." Institute of Science in Society (November 3, 2001). http://www.i-sis.org.uk/FoodborneIllnesses.php

70. Ibid.

Chapter 3: Connect These Dots

1. Suzuki, David. "Biotechnology: A Geneticist's Personal Perspective." http://www.davidsuzuki.org/files/general/dtsbiotech.pdf

2. "Labeling Issues, Revolving Doors, rBGH, Bribery and Monsanto." SourceWatch, Center for Media and Democracy (2007). http://www.sourcewatch.org/index.php?title=Labeling_Issues%2C_Revolving_Doors%2C_rBGH%2C_Bribery_and_Monsanto

3. Tarleton, John. "USA: Bush Delivers Emergency AIDS Relief to Republican Allies." CorpWatch (July 2, 2003).http://www.corpwatch.org/article.php?id=7488

4. Cummings, Claire Hope. "Trespass." Mindfully.org, originally published in *World Watch Magazine* (January-February 2005). http://www.mindfully.org/GE/2005/Trespass-Genetic-Engineering1jan05.htm

5. Ibid.

6. St. Clair, Jeffrey. "The Monsanto Machine." Common Dreams, originally released by *In These Times* (March 7, 1999). http://www.commondreams.org/headlines/090300-03.htm

7. "President Bush Urges Congress to Pass BioShield Legislation." Remarks by the President at the BIO 2003 Convention Center and Exhibition, Washington, D.C. Office of the Press Secretary (June 23, 2003). http://www.whitehouse.gov/news/releases/2003/06/20030623-2.html

8. Brown, Elizabeth. "More than 2,000 Spin Through Revolving Door." The Center for Public Integrity (April 7, 2005). http://www.publicintegrity.org/lobby/report.aspx?aid=678

9. Hightower, Jim. "Representing The Real America." *Hightower Lowdown* (July 24, 2007) http://jimhightower.com/node/6172.

10. Gettelman, Elizabeth. "The K(a-ching!) Street Congressmen." *Mother Jones* (November-December 2004) p. 24.

11. St. Clair, Jeffrey. "The Monsanto Machine." Common Dreams, originally released by *In These Times* (March 7, 1999). http://www.commondreams.org/headlines/090300-03.htm

12. Cohen, Robert. "Report on FDA Lawsuit on rBGH." *Not Milk* Newsletter (January 3, 1999). http://www.notmilk.com/deb/010399.html

13. Cohen, Robert. "Bush & Monsanto: Today's Pelican Brief." Alkalize for Health, originally released in the *Not Milk* Newsletter (March 18, 2001). http://www.alkalizeforhealth.net/Lbushmonsanto.htm

14. "Labeling Issues, Revolving Doors, rBGH, Bribery and Monsanto." SourceWatch, Center for Media and Democracy (2007). http://www.sourcewatch.org/index.php?title=Labeling_Issues%2C_Revolving_Doors%2C_rBGH%2C_Bribery_and_Monsanto

15. Ibid.

16. Christiansen, Andrew. "Recombinant Bovine Growth Hormone: Alarming Tests, Unfounded Approval." Mindfully.org, originally released as Rural Education Action Project, Vermont (July 1995). http://www.mindfully.org/GE/RBGH-Alarming-TestsJul95.htm

17. "Consumer Federation of America." SourceWatch (2005). http://www.sourcewatch.org/index.php?title=Consumer_Federation_of_America

18. "Monsanto Hijacks Safe Food Coalition." PR Watch, Center for Media and Democracy (2005). http://www.prwatch.org/prwissues/1994Q3/monsanto.html

19. Ibid.

20. St. Clair, Jeffrey. "The Monsanto Machine." Common Dreams, originally released by *In These Times* (March 7, 1999). http://www.commondreams.org/headlines/090300-03.htm

21. "About Robert T. Fraley." Biotechnology Industry Organization (June 16, 2004). http://www.bio.org/events/2004/media/brunch/fraley.asp

22. St. Clair, Jeffrey. "The Monsanto Machine." Common Dreams, originally released by *In These Times* (March 7, 1999). http://www.commondreams.org/headlines/090300-03.htm

23. "Profile: L. Val Giddings." GM Watch (2007). http://www.gmwatch.org/profile1.asp?PrId=51

24. "Sippel, Rodney W." Edmonds Institute (2004). http://www.edmonds-institute.org/html/directory-98.html

25. Barboza, David. "Bias Issue Arises for Monsanto Case Judge." *New York Times* (January 9, 2004). http://query.nytimes.com/gst/health/article-printpage.html?res=950CE1DB1F31F93AA35752C0A9629C8B63

26. "Hale, Marcia." Edmonds Institute (2005). http://www.edmonds-institute.org/html/directory-45.html

27. "IPC Funding and Donors." International Food & Agricultural Trade Policy Council (2006). http://www.agritrade.org/about/funding.html

28. Nichols, John. "Now Bush is Picking on Kids." *The Nation* (March 27, 2005). http://www.thenation.com/blogs/thebeat?bid=1&pid=2289

29. "Monsanto's High Level Connections to the Bush Administration." SourceWatch, Center for Media and Democracy (2005). http://www.sourcewatch.org/index.php?title=Monsanto%27s_High_Level_Connections_to_the_Bush_Administration

30. Ibid.

31. Supreme Court of the United States. *The Justices of the Supreme Court.* (2005). http://www.supremecourtus.gov/about/biographiescurrent.pdf

32. "Fisher, Linda J." Edmonds Institute (2004). http://edmonds-institute.org/html/directory-32.html

33. Spitzer, Skip. "Corporate Power." Network of Concerned Farmers, originally released by FinancialExpress.com (September 16, 2005). http://www.non-gm-farmers.com/news_details.asp?ID=2428

34. Lambrecht, Bill & Shesgreen, Dierdre. "Monsanto Continues to Block Federal Legislation on Labeling & Safety Testing of GE Foods & Crops." Organic Consumers Association (September 12, 2005). http://www.organicconsumers.org/monsanto/safety091305.cfm

35. Laskow, Sarah. "State Lobbying Becomes Billion-Dollar Business." The Center for Public Integrity (December 20, 2006). http://www.publicintegrity.org/hiredguns/report.aspx?aid=835

36. Ismail, M. Asif. "Breaking the Law: At Least One in Five Companies Lobbying Fail to File Required Forms." The Center for Public Integrity (April 7, 2005). http://www.publicintegrity.org/lobby/report.aspx?aid=676

37. "Biotechnology Industry Organization." Capital Eye, Center for Responsive Politics (2005). http://www.capitaleye.org/bio-BIO.asp

38. "BIO Board of Directors." Biotechnology Industry Organization (2005). http://www.bio.org/speeches/pubs/milestone05/board.asp

39. Bleifuss, Joel. "No Small Genetic Potatoes." Earthsave.org, originally released by *In These Times* (January 10, 2000). http://boston.earthsave.org/NoSmallgeneticPotatoes.htm

40. "Utility Patents Held by U.S. Government, Federal, and State by Technology Class and Subclass." Economic Research Service, USDA (2005). http://www.ers.usda.gov/data/AgBiotechIP/

41. "Facts about Federal R&D." RaDiUS Research and Development Database (2005). https://radius.rand.org/radius/federal_rd.html

42. Lehne, Richard & van Roozendaal, Gerda. "U.S. Government Role in Biotechnology R&D." *Biotechnology and Development Monitor* (September 1995). http://www.biotech-monitor.nl/2403.htm

43. Ibid.

44. "About Us." Agricultural Biotechnology Communicators (2002). http://agribiotech.info/AboutUs.htm

45. Fossum, Donna, Painter, Lawrence S., Eisman, Elisa, Ettedgui, Emile, & Adamson, David M. *Vital Assets: Federal Investment in Research and Development at the Nation's Universities and Colleges.* (2004). http://www.rand.org/pubs/monograph_reports/2005/MR1824.pdf

46. "Biotechnology in the Midwest." American Chemical Society, *Chemical & Engineering News* (February 23, 2004). http://pubs.acs.org/cen/employment/8208/8208employment.html

47. McGeary, Michael & Smith, Philip. *State Government Initiatives in Biotechnology.* Biotechnology Industry Organization Report The Lasker Foundation (October 26, 2001). http://www.laskerfoundation.org/ffpages/reports/m11.htm

48. Lehne, Richard & van Roozendaal, Gerda. "U.S. Government Role in Biotechnology R&D." Biotechnology and Development Monitor (September 1995). http://www.biotech-monitor.nl/2403.htm

49. Cline, Ned. "Biotech Center Breathes Life into State's Economy." *Business North Carolina* (September 1, 2003). http://www.highbeam.com/doc/1G1-108115571.html

50. Ibid.

51. Violino, Bob. "Strategic Insights." BIO-IT World (June 2003). http://www.bio-itworld.com/archive/061503/insights_midatlantic.html

52. Bantz, Sarah. "University Research & Genetic Engineering in the Midwest." *Z Magazine* (July-August 2002). http://www.zmag.org/ZMag/articles/julaug02bantz.html

53. Wirtz, Ronald A. "Come Hither, Biotech." Federal Reserve Bank of Minneapolis *FedGazette* (September 2003). http://minneapolisfed.org/pubs/fedgaz/03-09/biotech.cfm

54. Bantz, Sarah. "University Research & Genetic Engineering in the Midwest." *Z Magazine* (July-August 2002). http://www.zmag.org/ZMag/articles/julaug02bantz.html

55. Stamborsky, Al. "Monsanto Likely Will Base Subsidiary Here, CEO Says." (May 14, 2000). Biotech-info.net, originally released by St. Louis Post-Dispatch. http://www.biotech-info.net/subsidiary.html

56. Bantz, Sarah. "University Research & Genetic Engineering in the Midwest." *Z Magazine* (July-August 2002). http://www.zmag.org/ZMag/articles/julaug02bantz.html

57. "How to Lose Money on the Farm." Organic Consumers Association, *Organic Bytes* (October 7, 2002). http://www.organicconsumers.org/bytes/100702.cfm

58. "Wealthy Agribusinesses Continue to Collect the Bulk of Taxpayer Subsidies, Hurting Small Farms." Environmental Working Group (2005). http://www.ewg.org/news/story.php?id=4384

59. Dean, Stacy & Rosenbaum, Dorothy. "House Agriculture Committee Reconciliation Package Targets Food Stamp Program for Cuts." Center on Budget and Policy Priorities (November 8, 2005). http://www.cbpp.org/10-27-05fa.htm

60. Lochhead, Carolyn. "Pelosi Takes Heat for OK of Farm Bill." Common Dreams, originally released in the *San Francisco Chronicle* (July 17, 2007). http://www.commondreams.org/archive/2007/07/21/2676/

61. "Wealthy Agribusinesses Continue to Collect the Bulk of Taxpayer Subsidies, Hurting Small Farms." Environmental Working Group (2005). http://www.ewg.org/news/story.php?id=4384

62. Campbell, Dan. "Riceland's Richard Bell Retires in Year of Record Sales, Income." *USDA News Line* (September 2004). http://www.rurdev.usda.gov/rbs/pub/sep04/newsline.htm

63. "Riceland Completes Trade with Iraq." *USDA NewsLine* (2000). http://www.rurdev.usda.gov/rbs/pub/sep00/news.htm

64. "Fact sheet: Food Aid in the New Millennium—Genetically Engineered Food and Foreign Assistance." Food First, Institute for Food and Development Policy (2000). http://www.foodfirst.org/node/304

65. Campbell, Dan. "Riceland's Richard Bell Retires in Year of Record Sales, Income." *USDA News Line* (September 2004). http://www.rurdev.usda.gov/rbs/pub/sep04/newsline.htm

66. "Dairy Program Subsidies in the United States." Environmental Working Group Farm Subsidy Database (2005). http://www.ewg.org/farm/progdetail.php?fips=00000&progcode=dairy

67. Barrionuevo, Alexei. "Vicious Cycle of Subsidies and Overproduction." Organic Consumers Association, originally released by the *New York Times* (November 9, 2005). http://www.organicconsumers.org/ofgu/subsidies2.cfm

68. Ibid.

69. "USAID and GM Food Aid." Greenpeace International (October 2002). http://www.greenpeace.org.uk/MultimediaFiles/Live/FullReport/5243.pdf

70. Ibid.

71. "Diplomacy: The State Department at Work." U.S. Department of State, Bureau of Public Affairs (July 2001). http://www.state.gov/r/pa/ei/rls/dos/4078.htm

72. "About USAID." USAID (2005). http://www.usaid.gov/about_usaid/

73. "Profile, USAID—U.S. Agency for International Development." GM Watch (2005). http://www.gmwatch.org/profile1.asp?PrId=165&page=U

74. "Iraq's New Patent Law: A Declaration of War Against Farmers." *Focus on the Global South* and *GRAIN* (October 2004). http://www.grain.org/articles/?id=6

75. Tarleton, John. "USA: Bush Delivers Emergency AIDS Relief to Republican Allies." CorpWatch (July 3, 2003). http://www.corpwatch.org/article.php?id=7488

76. "The U.S. Assault on Biosafety—The WTO Dispute on GMOs." Greenpeace (December 2, 2005). http://www.greenpeace.org/international/press/reports/the-us-assault-on-biosafety

77. "Greenpeace Dismisses WTO Ruling and Predicts Europe Will Stay Closed to GMOs." Greenpeace International (February 7, 2006). http://www.greenpeace.org/international/press/releases/WTOruling060207

78. Vidal, John. "America's Masterplan is To Force GM Food on the World." *The Guardian* (February 13, 2006). http://www.guardian.co.uk/comment/story/0,1708257,00.html

79. Cummins, Ronnie. & Lilliston, Ben. *Genetically Engineered Food*, pp. 110-111. New York, NY: Marlowe & Company, 2004.

80. *Public Perceptions of Genetically Modified Foods: A National Study of American Knowledge and Opinion.* Food Policy Institute. Rutgers University, New Jersey (2003). http://www.foodpolicyinstitute.org/docs/reports/National Study2003.pdf

81. Pew AgBiotech Legislation Tracker 2001/2002. Pew Initiative on Food and Biotechnology (2001-2006). http://pewagbiotech.org/resources/factsheets/legislation/.

82. Lambrecht, Bill. "Monsanto Battles Effort to Require Labeling of Genetically Engineered Foods." CropChoice, originally released in the *St. Louis Post-Dispatch* (September 19, 2002). http://www.cropchoice.com/leadstryb 23b.html?recid=985

83. Ibid.

84. Ibid.

85. Bailey, Britt & Tokar, Brian. "Ag Industry Aims to Strip Local Control of Food Supplies: Big Food Strikes Back." CounterPunch.org. (May 26, 2005). http://counterpunch.org/tokar05262005.html

86. Ibid.

87. Hentoff, Nicholas & Silverglate, Harvey. *Writing Creative Nonfiction,* p. 148. Story Press, Cincinnati Ohio, 2001.

88. Collins, Ronald K. L., & McMasters, Paul. "Veggie-Libel Law Still Poses a Threat." Center for Science in the Public Interest, originally published in *Legal Times* (March 23, 1998). http://www.cspinet.org/foodspeak/oped/candm.htm

89. "SLAPP Happy: Corporations That Sue to Shut You Up." Center for Media and Democracy, PR Watch.org (Second Quarter 1997, Vol 4, No. 2). http://www.prwatch.org/prwissues/1997Q2/slapp.html

90. "Multi-Billion $$ Monsanto Sues More Family Farmers." Organic Consumers Association (2006). http://www.organicconsumers.org/monlink.cfm#farmers

91. Winters, Craig. "USDA Inspector General Blasts Regulation of Biotech Crops." The Campaign (January 1, 2006). http://www.thecampaign.org/weblog/?p=9

92. *Animal and Plant Health Inspection Service Controls over Issuance of Genetically Engineered Organism Release Permits.* U.S. Department of Agriculture Audit Report. (December 2005). www.thecampaign.org/USDA_IG_1205.pdf

93. *Seeds of Doubt: North American Farmers' Experiences of GM Crops.* The Soil Association (2002), p. 5. PDF available from Greenpeace.org. http://www.greenpeace.org/raw/content/international/press/reports/seeds-of-doubt-north-american.pdf

94. "U.S. Government Regulation." Biotechnology Industry Organization (2005). http://www.bio.org/foodag/action/fact3.asp

95. Currinder, Marian. "Private Sector Shaping Public Policy." OpenSecrets.org, Capital Eye Newsletter (September 1997). http://www.opensecrets.org/newsletter/ce45/ce45.01.htm

96. Olsson, Karen. "Ghostwriting the Law." *Mother Jones* (September-October 2002). http://www.motherjones.com/news/outfront/2002/09/ma_95_01.html

97. Bailey, Britt & Tokar, Brian. "Ag Industry Aims to Strip Local Control of Food Supplies: Big Food Strikes Back." CounterPunch.org. (May 26, 2005). http://counterpunch.org/tokar05262005.html

98. 2005 Seed & Plant Law Preemption Tracker. Environmental Commons (2005). http://www.environmentalcommons.org/gmo-tracker.html

99. "American Legislative Exchange Council." Center for Media & Democracy's SourceWatch (2007). http://www.sourcewatch.org/index.php?title= American_Legislative_Exchange_Council

100. Olsson, Karen. "Ghostwriting the Law." *Mother Jones* (September-October 2002). http://www.motherjones.com/news/outfront/2002/09/ma_95_01.html

Chapter 4: Biotech Persuaders

1. Barstow, David & Stein, Robin. "Under Bush, a New Age of Prepackaged Television News." Truthout.org, originally released in the *New York Times* (March 13, 2005). http://www.truthout.org/cgi-bin/artman/exec/view.cgi/37/9592

2. Whitehead, Susan. "New Biotech Propaganda Targets Children." Mindfully.org, originally released in *Peace & Freedom* (2001). http://www.mindfully.org/GE/GE3/Propaganda-Targets-Children-WILPF.htm

3. Cohen, Mitchel. "Monsanto Pushes Hormones on School Kids in their Milk." Mercola.com, originally released in Gary Null's *Natural Living* (August 2001). http://www.mercola.com/2001/aug/25/milk3.htm

4. Trueman, Kerry. "How Low Can Monsanto Go?" *The Huffington Post* (April 25, 2007). http://www.huffingtonpost.com/kerry-trueman/how-low-can-monsanto-go_b_46846.html

5. Mokhiber, Russell & Weissman, Robert. "The Ecologist and Monsanto." *Z Magazine* (1998). http://www.zmag.org/CrisesCurEvts/monsant.htm

6. Rampton, Sheldon & Stauber, John. *Trust Us, We're Experts: How Industry Manipulates Science and Gambles with Your Future*, p. 10. New York, NY: Tarcher/Putnam, 2001.

7. "Profile, Hudson Institute." GM Watch (2005). http://www.gmwatch.org/profile1.asp?PrId=59

8. "Cornucopia Institute Slams Monsanto Front Group for Spreading Disinformation on rBGH." Organic Consumers Association, originally released in *The Oregonian* (March 25, 2005). http://www.organicconsumers.org/rBGH/disinfo32905.cfm

9. "Leading Advocates Against Genetically Modified rBGH Milk File Citizens' Petition with FDA." The Campaign, originally released by PRNewswire-USNewswire (February 21, 2007). http://www.thecampaign.org/forums/showthread.php?t=519

10. Cohen, Mitchel. "Got Pus? Bovine Growth Hormone, Genetic Engineering and the New World Order." Mindfully.org. (August 13, 2001). http://www.mindfully.org/GE/GE3/rBGH-Got-Pus.htm

11. Kastel, Mark. "Down on the Farm: The Real rBGH Story Animal Health Problems, Financial Troubles." Mindfully.org (1995). http://www.mindfully.org/GE/Down-On-The-Farm-BGH1995.htm

12. Javers, Eamon. "Pro-Biotech Columnist Caught Taking Monsanto Money." Organic Consumers Association, originally released in *Business Week* Online (January 13, 2006). http://www.organicconsumers.org/ge/columnist011606.cfm

13. "rBGH Milk is rBHG Milk." Organic Consumers Association, *Organic Bytes #50* (February 11, 2005). http://www.organicconsumers.org/bytes/021105.cfm

14. "About the International Food Information Council (IFIC) Foundation." International Food Information Council (June 2007). http://ific.org/about/index.cfm

15. "International Food Information Council." SourceWatch (2005). http://www.sourcewatch.org/index.php?title=International_Food_Information_Council

16. Rampton, Sheldon & Stauber, John. *Trust Us, We're Experts: How Industry Manipulates Science and Gambles with Your Future*, p. 53. New York, NY: Tarcher/Putnam, 2001.

17. Ibid., p. 55.

18. "Profile: National Center for Food and Agriculture Policy (NCFAP)." GM Watch (2004). http://www.gmwatch.org/profile1.asp?PrId=94

19. "CropLife America." SourceWatch (2005) http://www.sourcewatch.org/index.php?title=CropLife_America

20. "American Council on Science and Health." SourceWatch (2005). http://www.sourcewatch.org/index.php?title=American_Council_on_Science_and_Health

21. Ibid.

22. Montague, Peter. "Lies in Defense of Humanism." *Rachel's Environment & Health Weekly #534* (February 20, 2007). http://www.rachel.org/bulletin/index.cfm?issue_ID=589

23. "Profile: Congress of Racial Equality (CORE)." GM Watch (2005). http://www.gmwatch.org/profile1.asp?PrId=174

24. "Bt Cotton in Makhathini, South Africa: The Success Story that Never Was." *GRAIN* (May 26, 2005). http://www.grain.org/nfg/?id=319

25. "About Biotechnology & Food." Compititive Enterprise Institute (2007). http://www.cei.org/sections/subsection.cfm?section=17

26. Mokhiber, Russell & Weissman, Robert. "Who Owns the Consumers Lobby?" *Mother Jones* (June 9, 2000). http://www.motherjones.com/news/feature/2000/06/fotc28.html

27. Gillam, Carey. (March 16, 2004). "U.S. State Department Promotes Biotech, Garners Critics." Planet Ark (March 16, 2004). http://www.planetark.com/dailynewsstory.cfm/newsid/24290/story.htm

28. Ibid.

29. Barstow, David & Stein, Robin. "Under Bush, a New Age of Prepackaged Television News." Truthout.org, originally released in the *New York Times* (March 13, 2005). http://www.truthout.org/cgi-bin/artman/exec/view.cgi/37/9592

30. Farsetta, Diane. "A Bumper Crop of Government-Produced News: The USDA's Broadcast Media and Technology Center." PR Watch, originally released in Trade Observatory (April 25, 2005). http://www.tradeobservatory.org/headlines.cfm?reflD=72770

31. Barstow, David & Stein, Robin. "Under Bush, a New Age of Prepackaged Television News." Truthout.org, originally released in the *New York Times* (March 13, 2005). http://www.truthout.org/cgi-bin/artman/exec/view.cgi/37/9592

32. Ibid.

33. Ibid.

34. Ibid.

35. Santa Ana, Rod. "New PBS Series to Feature Valley Agriculture." AgNews News and Public Affairs (March 11, 2005). http://agnews.tamu.edu/dailynews/stories/SOIL/Mar1105a.htm

36. Wasserman, Jim. "America's Heartland: KVIE and American Public Television Show Criticized Over Its Sponsors." Sacramento Bee (July 26, 2005). http://www.mindfully.org/Industry/2005/Americasheartland.orgTV26jul05.htm

37. Getzan, Christopher. "Monsanto-Sponsored PBS Documentary Riles Small Farming Advocates." Organic Consumers Association (August 24, 2005). http://www.organicconsumers.org/monsanto/pbs082405.cfm.

38. Ibid.

39. "More on Monsanto & PBS's New Partnership; Monsanto Takes Over America's Heartland." Organic Consumers Association (June 16, 2005). http://www.organicconsumers.org/monsanto/morepbs061605.cfm

40. Ibid.

41. Santa Ana, Rod. "New PBS Series to Feature Valley Agriculture." AgNews News and Public Affairs (March 11, 2005). http://agnews.tamu.edu/dailynews/stories/SOIL/Mar1105a.htm

42. "About Agriculture in the Classroom." Agriculture in the Classroom (AITC) (2006). http://www.agclassroom.org/aitc/index.htm

43. "Reading, Writing and Roundup Ready."PR Watch, Center for Media and Democracy (June 23, 2004). http://www.prwatch.org/taxonomy/term/87/9?page=3&from=10

44. *Your World: Biotechnology and You.* "Genetically Modified Food Crops" issue. Vol. 10, Issue No. 1. Biotechnology Institute. www.biotechinstitute.org/resources/pdf/yw10_1.pdf

45. Whitehead, Susan. "New Biotech Propaganda Targets Children." Mindfully.org, originally released by *Peace & Freedom* (2001). http://www.mindfully.org/GE/GE3/Propaganda-Targets-Children-WILPF.htm

Chapter 5: Take It Personally

1. "Primary Suspects: Ingredients and Products to Check." Mothers for Natural Law, Safe Food Campaign (2001). http://www.safe-food.org/-consumer/shop.html

2. "Barbara Boxer Introduces Bill for Mandatory Labeling of GE Foods in the US Senate." Organic Consumers Association (February 8, 2000). http://www.organicconsumers.org/ge/boxergebill.cfm

3. "Announcing: April 8th, Joint International GM Opposition Day." GM Watch (February 15, 2006). http://www.gmwatch.org/archive2.asp?arcid=6255

4. Ibid.

5. "Straus Organic Creamery Takes Bold Step to Prevent GMO Contamination." The Campaign, originally released by Strauss Family Creamery (March 6, 2007). http://www.thecampaign.org/forums/showthread.php?t=536

6. "Leading Organic & Natural Foods Retailer & Wholesale Distributor Will Test All Their Private Brand Labels for GMO Contamination." Organic Consumers Association, originally released by *Sustainable Food News* (March 9, 2007). http://www.organicconsumers.org/articles/article_4477.cfm

7. Buglass, Dan. "It's Rapidly Becoming an Organic World." Scotsman.com (July 28, 2007). http://business.scotsman.com/agriculture.cfm?id=1177602007

8. Ibid.

9. "Organic Farming Can Feed the World, U-M Study Shows." University of Michigan News Service (July 10, 2007). http://www.ns.umich.edu/htdocs/releases/story.php?id=5936

10. Ibid.

11. Roseboro, Ken. "FAO Looks at Organic Agriculture as Solution for Global Food Security." Healthy News Report, originally released by *The Organic and Non-GMO Report* (December 2006).

12. Higa, Teruo, & Parr, James. *Beneficial and Effective Microorganisms for a Sustainable Agriculture and Environment.* International Nature Farming Research Center, Atami, Japan (1994). http://www.agriton.nl/higa.html

13. Ibid.

14. Genetic Engineering Action Network (2007). www.geaction.org

978-0-595-45180-7
0-595-45180-2

CPSIA information can be obtained at www.ICGtesting.com
Printed in the USA
LVOW100545010812

292342LV00001B/4/A